Sorry I Loved You

Rev. Michielle DJ Beck, RM

with

Marcus A. Lindemann, MSW, CH

chipmunkapublishing

the mental health publisher

Published by

Chipmunkapublishing

PO Box 6872

Brentwood

Essex CM13 1ZT

United Kingdom

http://www.chipmunkapublishing.com

Chipmunkapublishing gratefully acknowledge the support of Arts Council England.

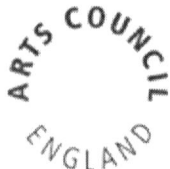

Dedication

For Smudo, Andy, Michi, and Thomas – your music gave me my life back, and helped me save my daughter as well. For the two of us, music really *is* therapy. You have been an integral part of what truly made me joyous again, and it is a debt which I can never repay. *Eure Musik läßt meine Seele wieder singen.*

- Michielle DJ Beck

To all the family and friends who I have been honored to share this life with – you have all taught me so many things, I would not be who I am without you. "If you take care of what you have, what you have will take care of you."

- Marcus A. Lindemann

Michielle DJ Beck with Marcus A. Lindemann

About the Author

Rev. Michielle DJ "Michi" Beck grew up in the desert southwest, and has been a professional freelance writer and editor since 1994. She has dealt with codependency, relationship addiction, depression, and anxiety all her life. With this book she brings the message that there is always hope for the future, no matter what the circumstances of the past have been – and there is time to be whole and happy again, all on your own. If anyone knows that, she does. Michi lives in Navarre, Florida.

You can visit her on the web at:
http://www.authormichibeck.blogspot.com.

About the Therapist

Marcus A. Lindemann, MSW, CH, graduated with a Masters of Clinical Social Work from the University of South Florida and specializes in the treatment of mood disorders, anxieties, post-traumatic stress, pain management, addiction, and codependence. An ordained Alakai in the order of Huna International, he has integrated a number of non-traditional therapy modalities in his work with clients for whom standard methods have been unsuccessful. He currently resides in Florida.

Michielle DJ Beck with Marcus A. Lindemann

Acknowledgments

Michielle DJ Beck would like to thank:

My mom and dad – I've finally learned that it's not about always agreeing with one another, but about respect in the face of differences. I'm proud of who I am today, and I could not have made it this far without your support and guidance.

My daughter, Andey – I'm so glad that where we are now is nothing like where we were then. It means everything knowing that you never gave up on me as a mother, as a friend, and as a human being, and I am blessed every day to have you in my life. Now we share not only our family ties but our *Freundschaft* as well.

The five men I married – you may not realize it, but you taught me more about who I was than I saw at the time. No matter what was said and done during our time together, I owe you thanks. I would not be who I am now without what I went through with you then.

The man I almost married – if it were not for you, I never would have heard the music that changed my life and brought me out of the darkness. The number of 'a-ha' moments I've had since I met you are too many to count, and I see more every day. I'll never forget that.

Marcus A. Lindemann – Thank you for the work you did to help bring this book to completion. Your professional insight and opinion at the end of each chapter, as well as your work on the foreword, added a valuable facet to this work that will undoubtedly help many people who struggle as I have struggled in the past.

My literary agent, Faye Swetky – I owe you a tremendous debt for simply believing in the merit of what I had to say, and recognizing that what I'd been through in my life could provide a benefit to others. Thank you.

D.J. Herda – I owe you profound thanks for your guidance and suggestions. If it were not for your advice on the structure and sections of the book, I may not have been able to offer my best work to the world and provide the help and healing so many people with addiction and codependency issues really need.

Marcus A. Lindemann would like to thank:

My parents and siblings – you have taught me what the words "family" and "love" really mean. That is and forever will be the greatest gift any man can receive.

My friends and teachers – I hope to be worthy of the love and knowledge you entrusted me with.

Michielle DJ Beck – thank you for this wonderful experience - and thank you for our ongoing friendship.

My Kahu Serge Kalihi King, Gloria King, Earl and Lois Stokes, Susan Pahinui Floyd, and my entire Huna International Ohana – Mahalo!

Ed Kaiwi – you are still very "special."

Foreword

When I was first asked whether I wanted to contribute to my friend's book my internal reaction was not favorable. What good would another self-help book on relationship addiction and codependence do? After all, several famous first-person accounts already exist - and many people have commented that, while those are helpful, they rarely go beyond the sharing of personal accounts. On the other hand, self-help manuals on codependence or relationship addiction oftentimes lack the personal stories that would make them more accessible to people. One type of book had too little information as to how to understand and deal with the problem in general, while the other lacked the personal insight of a fellow sufferer. Can you tell I was still rather biased?

I did not even wait until she had explained to me what she was actually planning before I passed my internal judgment. But when she made her case my interest was definitely piqued. What, she argued, could a book do that was based on the personal account of a relationship addict that had the professional assessment directly following the events? I was floored when I stopped to think about that. It was, in my opinion, a marvelous concept. People would be able to follow the life story, see the relationship addiction unfold, while at the same time being able to gain the understanding of how and why the events occurred. Not only that, a therapist's perspective would be able to point out both the foundations of the addiction and the means of how to undo those patterns. The reader would get the personal story and the treatment considerations all in the same process.

The more I thought about it, the more I liked the concept. What I did not expect was how the process of reading her account and then reflecting on it professionally would affect my own life. I am no stranger to codependency myself, but the level of self-evaluation this collaboration forced me to undertake was something that took me truly by surprise. Do not get me wrong, this is a good thing - a very good thing. It allowed me to improve on my own life as well as contribute to this work on a professional level. What better deal can anyone hope for than that? It also proved to me right then and there that this book would work. It would work well. I can only hope that those of you reading this will get as much out of my friend's personal account as I did.

Now what can the reader expect here? Well, first of all there is my friend's life story. No matter who you are, sharing one's own personal account of life takes a lot of guts, in my opinion. It is also a great way for personal healing, both for the one sharing it and the one it is shared with. At the end of each chapter I was privileged to add my professional reflection on what had transpired, usually a general explanation of the presented behavior patterns and where they come from.

That allows the entire book to be read in what I would call "easy chunks." Being an avid reader myself this makes the text very attractive to me, especially since I tend to have little personal time for reading these days. This is a book you can enjoy step-by-step. It may even be better that way. It allows us to read and then reflect, without having to get overwhelmed with too much information all at once.

You, dear reader, may find yourself in many of the described events. Others may be completely foreign to you. But through the entire account you will feel the honesty and sincerity of the unfolding story. I did. The reflections at the end of each chapter can then bridge those areas where the reader may not completely relate to the unfolding story, allowing for the discovery of underlying commonalities. The dedication and love that went into this project shines throughout. Of that much, I am sure. All in all, I would call the resulting book a wonderful opportunity for self-discovery and growth.

Above all, this text removes the specter of "abnormality" from terms like relationship addiction and codependence. These are not things that happen to just a select few. In here you will see just how widespread these conditions really are; how intrinsically "human" they are - and the reader can see that to suffer from any of these does not mean one is mentally damaged, stupid, or "wrong" in the greatest sense of the word. Relationship addiction and codependence can happen to anyone, even the most successful and brilliant of people. This book is not about pointing fingers. It is about self-realization and finding the means to overcome those things that keep us from being truly happy.

Do you think that might be worth taking this trip into my friend's life? I took that trip and in hindsight, I would not have missed it for the world.

-- Marcus A. Lindemann, MSW, CH

Introduction

I don't lie when people ask me my marital status. I'm brave enough to say I'm divorced. After all, it's much more common today and I'm no longer a social pariah. Really, though, my response is just a partial truth. I don't generally talk about how many times I've been married or offer that information unless I have no choice in the matter, or I find an important reason to do so. If it helps someone else I'll do it, even if it makes me uncomfortable. Otherwise, I'd rather not have people judge me, because they probably wouldn't understand and it takes too long to explain. When I'd been divorced only a couple of times it was still a little funny, and I found it easy to make jokes with other people who had also gotten married too young and realized they'd made a mistake – and there seemed to be a lot of us.

But after five failed marriages by the age of thirty-four, joking about my latest divorce lost its amusement value very quickly. And that didn't even consider the countless relationships that didn't go as far as the altar – everything from broken engagements to a couple of one-night stands. I'm not proud of the 'romantic' side of the social life I led for over twenty years, but there it is. Ignoring it won't make it go away. Talking about it here won't make it go away, either, but it might let someone else know that I (and a lot of other people) understand what he or she's dealing with.

If you're facing a lot of failed relationships – whether they're divorces or just break-ups – you're not alone in this. I promise. Ditto if you have poor, strained, or unhealthy relationships with co-workers, friends, or family members. There are more of us than you think, but we hide our pasts (and sometimes part of our present) a lot of the time because we're embarrassed. We're convinced that there's something 'wrong with us.' We ask ourselves why we're such screw-ups, why we can't do anything right, and why we don't feel like we have value and worth. The bottom line is that we aren't screw-ups. We have value and worth – to the people who care about us and to God. We do a lot of things right, we just spend too much time focused on the things we do wrong. Everyone makes mistakes, and when you're an addict, you tend to make the same ones, in the same area of life, over and over again until something helps you (or forces you) to break that pattern.

In my life, divorce wasn't the only issue. I wish I could say it was. I drank. I smoked. I didn't work very hard and couldn't hold a job. I panicked and shook and trembled and cried – a lot. And I hurt myself and sabotaged myself at every turn, for years. The worst part of it was that *I didn't know what was wrong with me.* All through my life, in the back of my mind, I'd wondered about that. What *was* wrong with me? I tried to get some help when I was young, but my parents were raised around the time of the Great Depression and I grew up in a time when mental health problems were still basically ignored – or even laughed at. You didn't ask for help, and you didn't spend money on 'mental health.' You sucked it up, and you dealt with it. There was nothing wrong with me. I just needed to 'get over it.' Except I couldn't. I just pretended to, and it made me unhappy, on the inside, for all those years.

It all started early – as early as I can remember – and it only got worse as I got older. Finally, after many long and confusing years I stumbled, completely by accident, onto a path of research and self-discovery, and today I can finally put a name to the main problem that has tormented me since my earliest memories: *I am a codependent relationship addict.* I didn't even know what that was when I came across the terms that make it up, and I didn't know there could be a lot more of my issues related to it. Have you ever had one of those moments where you see, hear, or read something, and all of a sudden you think "Holy cow! That's *ME!*"? Reading about codependency and relationship addiction gave me just that feeling. I remember thinking exactly that phrase. Well, maybe not *exactly* that phrase, but something pretty close to it, anyway.

Since that day, I have read virtually everything I've been able to find about codependency in its many forms, relationship addiction being only part of the equation. Unfortunately, I haven't seen anything that talks about what it's really *like*, all the way through, from a first-person account and from the heart. It's hard to get help from books and articles that don't – and can't – empathize with what you're dealing with. Clinical information is

14

good because it gives you background knowledge. I wouldn't discount it. If you have a condition, learn all you can about it - and be prepared for a lot of the information to conflict. Doctors don't know everything. They can't. When you hear someone who's been there, though, or when you read that person's words, that's when you really learn to start identifying with others, when you learn that there's hope, and when you know that you really aren't alone.

Chronicling something like this isn't always easy. There's a deep sense of shame that often comes along with it, and you usually try to put it in the past and forget about it. Those who are addicted to drugs or alcohol, they are pretty well understood today, and their addictions are seen as being valid and real by most of society. That doesn't make them less tragic or less severe – only better understood. But being 'addicted to love'? Well, that's just a song, isn't it? And what about being addicted to people-pleasing, addicted to worry, addicted to feeling nervous and afraid because it's the only thing you've ever really known, addicted to hurting yourself physically to make the emotional pain stop for just a little while, or addicted to having drama in your life?

Despite the lack of understanding that many people have about codependency, specifically as it relates to relationship addiction, it *is* real. There are a lot of people who have problems with it, but I suspect that many of them don't understand exactly what's wrong and how it can be addressed. They only know they are unhappy, and they think a relationship of some type will make them happy again. When it doesn't, they are lost. They think: "Well, I guess I just need a different relationship. That must be what's wrong!" So they leave their relationship, and they go and find another one, only to repeat the same pattern – a pattern which I finally succeeded in breaking, but only after many years, much effort, and a totally unexpected and unsolicited epiphany, which I promise I'll share with you in a later chapter.

Where I am now is somewhere that I'm very pleased with, even if I'm not particularly proud of how I got here. It was a long road. I want to tell you how I got here, and I intend to. It's an interesting and rather convoluted tale – funny in spots, sad in

15

others. But helpful, I believe. Tragic now, because I can look back over my shoulder at it and realize just how much I wish I would have known then what I know now. But we all wish that sometimes, don't we? When I think back on it, it's only then that I realize how much I actually went through, how many poor choices I made under the guise of finally hoping to 'get things right,' and how much of my life has been lived for other people and their dreams and ideals, instead of for myself. Where I am now isn't that place any more. Sometimes I fret and get depressed about all the time I 'wasted,' but if I wouldn't have gone through all of that, I wouldn't be where I am now, I wouldn't be able to help myself, and I wouldn't be able to help others. Not such a waste, really, when you look at it that way. There's value in every experience we go through as human beings, even when you can't see it at the time.

In order for what I've been through to be helpful to others I have to be willing to talk (or write) about it. That means *all* of it. The good and the bad. The things I'm ashamed of. The things I don't want to tell anyone because I'm still mortified by them. The things you might be going through right now when you think you're the only person in the world who could ever feel that way, ever have that kind of problem, or ever be 'that stupid.' Beating yourself up about the 'wrong choices' you've made, or the way you feel, or any problems you have or think you have won't help, but it's so very easy to do. I did it for a long time, and sometimes I still do – I just recognize it and control it better now. You can learn to do the same, no matter what kinds of addictions, codependency issues, or relationship problems you're facing, and no matter how long you've had them. Hope can never really die. It can only lie dormant for a while, and can always, *always* be resurrected by a willing heart and a gentle hand.

So I'm going to tell you about my life, and along the way I'm going to show you how you can learn to control yours, get yours back, or make yours even better. I won't be doing it through an 'I had it worse than you' sob story, but through honest, open truths about what I went through and why, and how I got better. The importance of the lesson won't be centered on the minute details of how I made changes, because everyone is different. What worked for me (mostly music, for starters) might not be something that matters much to you. Instead, the focus will be on the broader techniques that helped to improve life for me, and the techniques that can provide help and healing for so many codependent people.

These are techniques that can help you to get a handle on codependency, relationship addiction, sexual addiction, anxiety, depression, self-harm, and even drug and alcohol addiction if you take them to heart. These techniques are worth the time. More importantly, *you're* worth the time. It's easy to forget that when you're facing serious difficulties in your life, but I'm here to make sure you remember it again, even if it's been a long time – even if you weren't sure you ever knew it in the first place. To help me do that (and to help you get better), there will be a recap of what I did wrong and what to look for in your own life at the end of each chapter. I've enlisted the assistance of a wonderful professional who is also a close friend. He's going to weigh in on my experiences and information at the end of each chapter, as well. My hope is that he and I can convey to you the idea that, while healing might not always be easy, it's always worth the trouble. God bless. I wish you peace, joy, love, and contentment during your journey and forever after, but most of all I wish you freedom.

-- Michielle DJ Beck

Chapter 1: What I Know Now – And Why It Matters

My own journey with mental and emotional health issues actually began in childhood, although I didn't realize it until I was much older. It started, as most tales do, with parents. I thought my parents were amazing people. I still find them amazing in many ways, but my thoughts are now tempered with caveats that have come about from time, spiritual growth, and a deeper understanding of both of them - and of myself. I see people now for who they really are, as much as any of us are able to. It's one of the areas of growth that has been the most painful for me. I placed my parents – especially my father – on a pedestal when I was very young, like a lot of kids do, but I just never took them down as I got older. Finally taking them down has been difficult, but ultimately very rewarding. It has only been recently that I've been able to work through this, and I went through a lot of bad memories and failed relationships before I got to where I am now. But I got there, and so can anyone else who struggles with relationship addiction and/or codependency issues. It's not an easy journey, but it's definitely not an impossible one – and it's *very* worthwhile.

To really understand what happened to me, and what happens to other people who are codependent and/or relationship addicts, it's important to know what codependency and relationship addiction are and look at the different forms they can take. People who are codependents or relationship addicts can be addicted to (and struggle with) all different types of relationships. When most people think of these kinds of problems (if they think of them at all), they see them from the idea of one person who cannot seem to let go of a lost love, or from the idea of a stalker, obsessed with the neighbor down the street or the latest teen pop princess. These types of issues are only part of the group that make up codependents and relationship addicts. Here, you'll find that I mostly use the term 'relationship addiction' rather than 'codependency.' Even though it has such a close tie with codependency in general, many people don't recognize relationship addiction as a legitimate problem or see it as a true addiction – unless they or a loved one are facing it and are finally able to come to terms with the seriousness and significance of the problem. I want to change that, and struggling relationship addicts everywhere need the benefit of having their difficulties seen as real.

There are many types of relationship addicts, and often their problems do not seem obvious to the general public. The problems are there, however, lying just beneath the surface and manifesting themselves in different ways. That's what happened with me. I was never obsessed with a specific movie star, was never arrested for stalking anyone, and I certainly don't miss anyone I used to be involved with. I did, though, become what I termed a 'Serial Marrier,' in that I didn't think I could be 'Someone' without being 'Mrs. Someone Else.' Unfortunate, but not as uncommon as you might think.

If you read the more clinical books on relationship addiction, you'll find that most of them talk about codependency, too. For a long time, it was believed that codependency *was* relationship addiction, and there was no difference between the two. More recent information has shed light on the fact that, while many relationship addicts are codependent in some way, not all codependents are classified as relationship addicts. I am both codependent and a relationship addict, basically from my earliest memories. I can say that now, because I'm finally able to see it for what it is.

When I was in it, though, I never had it in any kind of realistic perspective. I think that's one of the real problems with relationship addicts, much like those who are addicted to drugs or alcohol. When you're right there in the middle of things, it seems normal to you. It's only when you start to get out of it, either through your own choices or through intervention from others, that you begin to realize just how far off 'normal' you actually were. You start to see that there are other options, and that most of society is not living the way you're living and feeling the way you're feeling. It shakes you up pretty badly at first, but it's worth it for what you get from the learning experience. You get the opportunity to take control of your own life once again instead of giving up control to an addiction, to other people, or both.

There are many different categories that relationship addicts fall under, and not everyone calls them relationship addicts. Some people call them 'love addicts,' of which relationship addicts are only a category. I prefer the term 'relationship addict,' but it's a personal preference. If the term 'love addict' works for you, use it. If you get a professional diagnosis, there are several designations you might fall under. It's important to know what they are, and how they're differentiated – but it's also important to understand that research into this issue will show discrepancies in how different people differentiate these groups. One person might list a particular trait as belonging to a particular type of addict, while another person might say that trait falls into another category entirely. Like physical medicine, mental health is not now, nor will it ever be, an exact science. There are always anomalies.

The definitions and explanations below are my personal thoughts and opinions on what I believe generally make up these categories, based on my understanding of what I've read and learned. They are probably not all inclusive, and other people might disagree with some of them. That's fine, as well. In addition, it's also important to understand that not everyone who engages in a particular behavior is an addict. Generally, addictions are similar to disorders in that they must affect one's life and daily functioning in order to be a concern, but this is not always obvious or accurate, and some people hide the reality of their life and what's taking place in it much better than others do.

These are my designations of relationship or love addiction, and what I feel they most commonly include. In looking at these, you can see how much of yourself you find in any or all of them. I know some of them make me feel like I'm looking in a mirror, but only if I'm really honest with myself.

- Relationship Addict – A relationship addict is a person who, like me, feels as though he or she has to be in a relationship to 'be someone.' This person is usually not addicted to a specific person, but only to the idea of a relationship, although some relationship addicts are addicted to the relationship they are in and will not leave their partner, even though they're often very unhappy. Some of these people feel they must 'rescue' their partner from something, and others feel they must be 'rescued,' so they look for someone to take care of them. I did both throughout my relationships, especially in my later marriages. My fourth marriage was to a man who had a nice house and a good job – someone to take care of me and my young daughter. My fifth marriage was to a man who was still very immature and needed a lot of emotional help and encouragement from others – someone I thought I could rescue.

The bottom line, though, was that neither one made me happy, and neither did the three marriages before that, and neither did the other relationships I was in when I was between marriages. I dated men who were much younger (trying to rescue them), and I dated men who were much (and I do mean *much*) older (trying to be rescued). Rescued from what, I still don't know. It didn't matter who I dated or married, though. I could have found someone who was actually as close to perfect as is humanly possible, and I still wouldn't have been happy. That's what a relationship addict *does*...he or she *has to have* a relationship. I thought I was nobody without a relationship. I loved the thrill of finding someone new, and the first kiss, and the first everything else. I wanted to get serious right away. I wanted commitment, a ring on my hand, a marriage certificate. But then I got bored with that person and moved on. Once the chase was over, I didn't necessarily like what I had caught.

It wasn't that the person was boring, either, but mostly that I was looking for a better relationship all the time. Someone new, someone exciting. Drama at its highest level. One of the most tragic issues with relationship addicts, though, is that they can be addicted to all kinds of relationships. It doesn't have to be their lover or their spouse. It can be an inability to let go of their children, or their parents, or a friend. Who would they be, if they weren't a parent or a child or a friend? Would they have any identity? Often, they don't think so. I know I didn't. Some relationship addicts will remain in a relationship even if it's extremely unhealthy for them, because they think they basically won't exist if they're alone, and they feel like they can't handle the change that comes along with that. I did that for a while, too.

- Obsessed Love Addict – Someone who's classified as an obsessed love addict finds that he or she is just that – obsessed. It doesn't matter if the object of the obsession is not available to the person, or if it's dangerous to be with that person. The obsessed love addict is interested only in the person he or she professes to 'love.' This is not actually love, of course, but an unhealthy attachment which needs to be broken. Many times, the obsessed love addict has never even met or spoken to the person he or she 'loves.' I was fortunate that I did not ever fall into this category, at least not severely. I did stay in relationships I knew were not good for me for a while, but in the end I got out of them, which is something many obsessed love addicts never find the ability to do. This can doom a person not only to a life of misery, but to actual physical harm if the person he or she is obsessed with is violent or dangerous.

All too often the battered women that you see, the ones who just keep going back to their husbands or boyfriends because they 'love them' and the man 'didn't mean to hurt them' and it was 'their fault for doing something stupid' and they 'deserved it,' are obsessed love addicts. They know, deep down, that things are not the way they really should be, but they tell themselves lies and they go on with their lives. Often they have children, so they stay 'for the sake of the kids,' not realizing all along how much damage they're doing to their children. Kids mimic what they see, and they try to be like their parents. Kids who see a mother who gets hit when she does something wrong are going to come to see that as normal, perpetuating a dangerous pattern when they get older and have relationships of their own.

- Sex Addict – This might seem pretty obvious, as many sex addicts go out and find one-night stands and other sexual situations such as hiring prostitutes or offering to pay others for sex. However, people who fall into this designation are not all addicted to sex in the way many individuals would assume. Some who have this problem may also watch excessive amounts of pornography or engage in frequent and/or aggressive masturbation, well beyond what is considered to be 'normal' for a person of their age and gender. For others, a combination of these behaviors may also be seen. Whether a person overindulges in himself or herself, or in other people – either through watching, participating, or both – he or she will generally be considered a sex addict if these sex-related behaviors affect his or her daily life.

There is, unfortunately, another type of sex addict – the rapist. Most rapists are interested in power over their victims, but there are also individuals who will rape because of their perceived 'need' for sex. They have a compulsion for it, and they must get their 'fix,' just as a cocaine addict must find more of the drug he or she feels unable to do without. A person with this strong a sexual compulsion can be dangerous to others, and is seriously in need of treatment. What is not realized, though, is how many other sex addicts, who would never rape someone, are still dangerous – both to themselves and others.

There are so many sexually-transmitted diseases today that sex addicts are often putting themselves at great risk, and they put their future partners at great risk, as well. It's one of the serious concerns with sex addiction that most people don't even think about, but it's very important that these individuals not only get help for their addiction but also take steps to protect themselves and others. They can pass dangerous and deadly diseases to a lot of people, sometimes before they even know they're infected. Education on this issue as well as education on sex addiction in general is the first step to helping many of the people in this category.

- Ambivalent Love Addict – The ambivalent love addicts are usually avoidant personalities. They really, desperately want to have loving relationships, but they're so afraid of emotional intimacy with others they often either avoid the relationships they want, or find some way to destroy them. These people are fine with letting go, but they have trouble moving forward from there. In other words, breaking up with a person is easy for them, because it stops them from getting intimate – and by 'intimate' I mean mentally and emotionally, not physically – but finding a new person and becoming intimate with that person is not something they're prepared for. They generally can only take a relationship to a certain level before they begin to feel trapped and start looking for ways to get away from the other person. They're commitment-phobic, and they usually have 'good excuses' as to why they broke up with someone.

I engaged in some of this early on, and even in my marriages this was a problem. I didn't have any trouble getting divorced, other than the shame and guilt of letting others (mostly my father) down. Emotionally, it really didn't bother me that much that my marriage was ending…sometimes I was even relieved, and excited to be 'getting rid' of this person. How cold, and cruel. I know. Some of the men I divorced didn't seem too bothered by it, which makes me think they might have been suffering from some of the same kinds of problem themselves, but others…I know of two ex-husbands who turned to alcohol (and one briefly to drugs, as well) after we split up. I broke their hearts – at least for a moment, and it took them time to recover. I don't say that out of some perverted sense of bragging rights, and I don't say it to sound like I'm some wonderful and perfect 'catch' they couldn't bear to let get away. I say it to provide a better understanding of some of the damage that relationship addiction can cause. I still feel bad about hurting them, even though I know in many ways it was not my fault, just like it was not their fault – it was just part of my addiction; my disease. We can only do what we can with what we have.

- Narcissistic Love Addict – Most of us have heard the term 'narcissist' used before, generally about someone who thinks he or she is 'really something.' For a narcissistic love addict, however, the goal is not about physical beauty, but about thwarting anyone who threatens their happiness in any way. They have a strong sense of entitlement, and they want to do what they want to do, regardless of how others feel about it. In short, they are bullies. And they are the worst kind of bullies, because they aren't secret cowards at heart, and they don't back down when you stand up to them. I was briefly involved with someone like this once. He was very controlling, and he didn't seem to think I would ever do anything about it. A narcissistic love addict believes he or she can do whatever feels right, and others must simply fall in line with that.

Thankfully, I never married this person. He was a police officer who shall remain nameless. He lived in a nice home, and the fact that I lived in a mobile home at the time wasn't good enough for him. He looked around my brand new and spotless mobile home with disdain and wrinkled his nose.

"A *trailer*? Don't you want something *better* out of life?" he asked with a sneer.

He cancelled dates, didn't show up when he said he would, and asked 'just what the hell was wrong with me' when I questioned anything or let him know I didn't like something he did. He refused sex, because he said he 'wasn't ready.' I respected that at first, but in hindsight I think it was another way of controlling me and our relationship. If I wanted to be physically intimate and he didn't then he had the upper hand, and another measure of control. Instead of being honest with him and telling him I didn't want to see him anymore, I finally just stopped calling him or taking his calls.

I was lucky, though, because he got tired of that and 'broke up with me' and left me alone. It was very early in the relationship, and when I look back on it, I'm glad I didn't date him any longer. Had I done that, he might not have let go so easily. He was a big guy, and he could be scary, and he carried a gun. Not someone I really wanted to piss off, but I wasn't going to become his doormat, either. Narcissistic love addicts can be *very* dangerous people. It's not their fault, really, but that doesn't make it any safer for the people they get involved with.

- Codependent Love Addict – The codependent love addict is the one most people think of, if they think of love addicts at all. A person might not know what the right term is for this kind of person, but he'll know this kind of relationship when he sees it. These are what I consider the 'generalized' relationship or love addicts. People who are codependent love addicts will do almost anything to keep the relationships they have. They'll put up with abuse and neglect, they'll go above and beyond the call of duty to please another person, and they'll sacrifice what they want, what they need, and *who they are* to keep another person in their life – and it doesn't have to be a spouse or a lover. Some people do this for parents, children, or friends.

There's nothing at all wrong with doing things for people. If that was the case, just about everyone on the planet would be a codependent love addict. However, you should only do things for people if you want to do those things and if they don't interfere with what you want for yourself. If you don't take care of yourself, you can't take care of anyone else – at least not in a healthy way. The self-sacrificing behavior usually doesn't work for long. The feelings of sadness and despair that accompany it come out in other ways. Some people drink, some yell at their children and their pets, some just go to an early grave because of the stress they're under. I firmly believe that, if I would have stayed married to my fifth ex-husband, I would have been dead within ten years – maybe fifteen if I was lucky. My family has pretty good longevity, but the stress of our marriage was taking its toll, and quickly. I married him for all the wrong reasons, and I felt both great relief (he's gone!) and great shame (can't I do *anything* right?) when our divorce was final. That last divorce was what pushed me toward a journey of self-discovery, but it wasn't quite enough to make me really understand and accept my codependency and relationship addiction issues. That would come later on.

- Saboteur – As the name implies, a saboteur will ruin relationships. He'll do this at whatever point he starts to feel frightened, and this can be different for everyone. For some people, it'll be when the idea of commitment begins to creep into the conversation, or when a commitment is about to take place (such as people who leave their fiancés at the altar, for example). For others, it'll be after sex for the first time with a new person. For still others, it might be much earlier – right after the first date, for example, or even before that date ever takes place. Every saboteur is different based on the point where he decides to destroy the relationship and how he chooses to go about that. I was guilty of some of this. I would find reasons to end relationships, and it was usually by finding a way to make the other person leave. On one occasion I believed I was totally justified in doing this, but in hindsight there were better ways to have handled it. I should have stood my ground and just told him to leave, but since my father didn't seem to think the guy had done anything wrong when he did what he did, I thought I had to make the guy leave me, so my father would blame him instead of me.

I didn't sabotage every relationship I ever had, but I did sabotage or try to ruin a fair number of them – mostly those with spouses or lovers. I have not tried to destroy my relationship with my parents or with my daughter, but those relationships have changed a lot as I've learned about myself and my addiction. If we can all get through that process, I think my relationships with them – and by extension everyone else – will be much healthier in the long run. The growth process, though, is never an easy one, and it seems to be this process the saboteur is most afraid of. These individuals are so frightened of valuing and committing to a relationship that they run so they don't have to change and grow. I'd be willing to bet that most of them don't even have any understanding of why they do this. I know for a long time I just told myself the person was bad for me, or a jerk, or it was his fault, etc. Only when I began to recover did I see what I had done to destroy the relationships with so many of these people.

- Torch Bearer – The torch bearer is the person who suffers from unrequited love. He might profess to be in love with a movie star, or with the person down the street. It really doesn't matter who the object of affection is, as long as that person is totally unavailable. There's some argument, though, about what 'totally unavailable' means. I think, for the most part, it involves being realistic. Technically, unless a person is deceased, he or she is not *totally* unavailable. Married people can get divorced, movie stars can meet 'normal' people, and stranger things have happened. However, I think in most instances someone who is married or someone who would be incredibly difficult to connect with through expected life circumstances would be considered to be 'totally unavailable.'

Carrying a torch for someone can be dangerous – and it's not the same as having a crush on someone. A torch bearer could potentially become so obsessed with a person that other parts of life – family, work, etc. – are neglected. Money could be spent to try to find the object of affection, and some torch bearers even become so angry or despondent when they find out their fantasy person has someone real in his or her life in a romantic sense that they either hurt themselves or another person. If you actually care about someone as a human being it's not about whether you have that person, it's about whether that person is happy. A torch bearer would find that to be a totally alien concept.

- Seductive Withholder – The seductive withholder is, to me, one of the easiest relationship addicts to understand, at least on a conceptual level. While most of us don't fall into the category of actually *being* a seductive withholder, I think most of us have practiced some of the traits of it from time to time. Anyone who has whispered sweet promises for later in her husband's ear to get him to get up and take out the trash has done something similar to what a seductive withholder would do – but for most people that innocent 'bribery' is harmless. For the true seductive withholder, however, sex and companionship are wonderful as long as he wants it. As soon as that person feels anxious, frightened, threatened, or otherwise upset, the affection in any form is withheld. It goes far beyond the normal play that most couples experience, or the angry wife who withholds sex for the night because her husband came home late after one too many drinks with his buddies.

Seductive withholders need to feel safe. As long as they do, they're freely affectionate with their partners. However, even a simple threat can cause problems for a person like this. These individuals also have a very repetitive pattern of this behavior, unlike the saboteur who will more than likely just end the relationship when threats appear on the horizon. These threats can come from very common or very small problems, but to a seductive withholder all problems are huge and serious. They can make mountains out of molehills, and they drag their partners along for the ride. A person who's a seductive withholder may also withhold other types of affection besides sex. For example, if a parent feels threatened in some way by a child (maybe a mother's daughter is smarter, prettier, etc.) the parent might be much less affectionate with that child, out of jealousy or fear. It's not only the romantic relationship that can be damaged by a seductive withholder.

- Romance Addict – The true romance addict isn't afraid to get involved with people and care about them very quickly, but the deep commitment that's needed for a full and lasting relationship isn't present. A romance addict is often confused with a sex addict, but most sex addicts have no interest in bonding with anyone at all. Instead, they simply want to gratify their urges. For the romance addict, the goal isn't sexual gratification, but emotional gratification – drama and love and whirlwind romance. These kinds of romances rarely last in the real world, though. They're mostly for the movies. Even the happiest of real-world couples occasionally fight or get tired of one another, if only briefly.

For the romance addict, multiple partners are important. There is no desire to commit to just a single person. These addicts get a type of 'high' off drama and romance, especially in the early stages of a relationship when everything is new and exciting. I've been guilty of this one in the past, as well. I never had a lot of multiple relationships going on, but I was definitely addicted to the high of that first glance, first touch, first kiss. It was intoxicating - and incredibly unhealthy. If it had been real love it would have been wonderful, but since it was only pseudo-love it didn't last, and neither did the relationship. Depressing, really, because most people want and need love in their lives. A romance addict doesn't know how to get these things in a healthy and mature way, and that's true of basically any kind of relationship or love addict, no matter how you define or designate them.

- Any and All Combinations of the Above – You've probably noticed that I 'admitted guilt' several times in the preceding discussion. Although I say I am codependent and a relationship addict, there is really more to it than that. I just use the term because it's simplified. Really, though, I am a relationship addict. I am a romance addict. I am a codependent love addict. I am a saboteur. I am these things now, just as I have been them in the past, and I will be them in the future. Now, though, I know about it, and I am taking what steps I can to keep it from manifesting itself.

You can experience recovery, and if you saw yourself in one or more of those descriptions, don't think you're beyond hope. You're not. You simply have work to do, and that work has to matter to you. If it doesn't, you won't get better. But when you get to the place where you *know* your life has to change, that's a great place to work from. Even commitment-phobic people can generally commit to their recovery from that place, because they're finally somewhere that allows them to see the value in themselves and in what they could make of their life.

I use the term 'relationship addict' as a generalization, by the way, so don't think that being diagnosed as a 'love addict' or a 'romance addict' means that this book won't help you or won't be relevant to what you're going through. While my life experience is much closer to some of the specific designations than to others, all addictions of this type have similarities. The goal here is not to diagnose the reader or to question a diagnosis that has already been made, either through therapy or through self-discovery. My own diagnosis has come through self-discovery and spiritual growth in the beginning, with later confirmation through a trained professional.

Truthfully, it doesn't matter how you come to a realization about codependency or relationship addiction. It only matters that you realize it. Once that takes place you can work toward understanding, and recovery can begin. If you realize through the reading of this book that you share my problems, you can get the help you need. If you've already been diagnosed in some other way and this book helps you, that's wonderful. If you're trying to help or better understand a loved one, you may find a lot of benefit in reading what I have to say. If you just like reading about what others have gone through, that's also fine. If I can bring any kind of help or healing to even one person through this book, everything I've gone through in the past will not have been wasted time.

If you're finding yourself with a lot of excuses and no real reasons today, maybe knowing you're not alone and learning about codependency and relationship addiction will help you get a better understanding of what you might need to do next. It might also help you – if you're codependent or a relationship addict yourself – not to feel so ashamed. One of the unfortunate stigmas that come along with the 'relationship addict' or 'codependent' label is a deep sense of shame. Society as a whole doesn't seem to see this as being a 'real' addiction.

When was the last time you heard about codependency or relationship addiction on the nightly news or saw it discussed in a magazine? I know I can't remember *ever* hearing about relationship addiction on the news, or seeing a study on it. Codependency is a more common term, but even that isn't talked about much. Researching the topic doesn't provide the kind of results that researching other types of addictions provides.

There are web sites out there that talk about it, but not in the kind of volume you would see with drug or alcohol addiction. There are some journal articles, too, and some clinical books, but most of them aren't that recent. Because people aren't told about it, they don't see it as real. They see it as a made-up problem, or another excuse that people use when they aren't smart enough know better, or when they refuse to own up to their own behavior. Those things are far from the truth, but they're how relationship addicts and codependents are often stereotyped. Naturally, shame comes with that. If you have a legitimate problem, and it has caused you to do things that other people think are bad, and you don't know why you do these things and can't seem to stop, it's only natural that you feel ashamed, but you don't have to feel that way anymore.

You might have asked yourself things like:

- What's wrong with me?
- Why can't I be happy with the person I am?
- Why can't I be happy with the person I have in my life? (This could be a parent, child, lover, friend, or anyone you have a relationship with.)
- Why do I make such 'stupid' choices?
- Why do I keep making the same mistakes over and over and over again?
- Why can't I have a 'normal' life?
- Am I the only one this is happening to?

I asked myself all those questions, too…and for the longest time, I had no answers. I didn't even really want to ask the questions; they were just there, popping up in my mind in the dead of night when I couldn't sleep yet again. I tried to push them away but they wouldn't leave, and they haunted me literally for years. As I got older I tried making the questions stop by actually answering them, but my 'answers' were generally just more excuses.

Addictions are insidious creatures. They sneak into your life and slowly steal it away from you, and you don't realize they're there, or the kind of damage they're doing, usually until you hit rock bottom. Some of us are lucky – we don't have to completely bottom out before realizing we have a problem that has to be solved. Instead, we may have a grand epiphany, an 'a-ha moment,' that brings us to an understanding of what the real issue is. This doesn't happen to everyone, and if it hasn't happened to you that certainly doesn't mean you can't get help and be successful at conquering your addiction. Those a-ha moments often come when you're least looking for them. You may have one yet, or you may recover without some type of epiphany. Everyone is different, and it's not always a good idea to compare your speed and details of recovery to someone else. They have their own race to run, so don't worry about them. Worry about and focus on yourself and what you need to address for your own personal recovery.

Like any other type of addiction, relationship addiction is always going to be there. The goal is not to 'cure' it, because that really doesn't happen. The goal is to understand it, and control it – instead of letting it control you. It can be done. I'm living proof. But anyone who thinks it's easy has never really been through it. It's similar to the panic attacks which are also a part of my life, in that a person who has never experienced one really cannot have a complete understanding of what it feels like. The same is true for almost any experience in life. Even people who've been through the same thing might still have experienced it differently. The idea that you 'know how someone feels' is an illusion most people suffer from. While we might have an idea of what someone else has been through, our perception and theirs are never really the same.

What I Did Wrong
- I put the needs of others before my own needs, even when I knew it wasn't the right path for me.
- I let my fear over what others would think of me control how I lived my life.

34

- I didn't learn from my mistakes until I had made them repeatedly.
- I kept forcing myself to do what I thought I should do to 'fit in' with society's norms.
- I wasn't willing to face my issues and work on them even though I knew that there was something 'not right.'
- I was too proud to seek any kind of help, but at the same time I didn't think I was worth the effort.
- I didn't talk to the people closest to me, openly and honestly, and tell them what I was feeling and thinking so they could help me.

What To Look For
- Feeling uncomfortable because what you *believe* about your life isn't fitting the facts – it's called 'cognitive dissonance.'
- Doing things *only* to please someone else with no regard to how you actually feel about those things.
- Anything in your life that fits into one or more of the 'relationship addiction' categories I've talked about in this chapter.
- An inability to be happy if you're not in a relationship with a spouse or lover.
- Not being happy if things are actually going all right for once – in other words, not being happy if you don't have some kind of drama going on in your life.
- Using drugs or alcohol or other coping mechanisms to hide what's really going on with your life and/or your dissatisfaction with it.
- An unwillingness to talk to anyone and admit you're having a problem – and it doesn't have to be a therapist. It can be a trusted friend, a family member, a 1-800 hotline, or anyone you can confide in so you can face your problems and start healing.
- Running from your past instead of using what you've been through to secure a better future for yourself.

What the Therapist Says

There is an old saying that self-discovery is the first step toward betterment. Despite its cliché nature that saying does bear true a lot of times. In order to improve ourselves we must first have an idea what needs to be improved upon. Sadly, as far as relationships are concerned our ability to do just that is often hampered by our own attitudes. Many people believe their innermost values come from conscious personal choice. Yet, in reality, many of our most deeply held beliefs derive directly from our upbringing. We mimic what we believe is a "good" or a "bad" relationship by what we see our parents do and by what society tells us is "right," "good," and "needed." This usually happens without us being aware of it. The way we feel about matters of the heart is something that does not require a lot of conscious effort. The easiest way to prove that is by looking at how we judge people who have different levels of "success" in relationships. We will evaluate someone who is divorced or single differently from a person who is not. An individual who has been in a successful relationship for a while is ascribed a different value by us than someone who has had a number of failed relationships. Again, we do not think about this consciously. It just happens, whether we have a relationship and its degree of success is definitely a factor in how we ascribe worth to a person and ourselves.

How does all of this relate to the term "codependence"? There are a number of different definitions to this term and many professionals hold their own opinions as to which one is correct. To me, codependence defines a personality trait - a very deeply-held set of attitudes within an individual's subconscious mind. Note that this is different from my definition of "addiction," which describes a behavior pattern, as discussed later. People who suffer from codependence usually suffer from an underdeveloped sense of self or self-worth. One of the most obvious signs of that is when a person considers himself or herself innately worthless without some sort of interaction with other people. A codependent individual requires continuous feedback from an outside source in order to feel "worthwhile" or "whole."

A codependent's sense of self depends on something that is not part of him. This need for outside validation will often cause such an individual to engage in behaviors that supply this validation. The list of behaviors this can include is vast, the more well-known including alcoholism, drug abuse, gambling, and other addictions. Yet codependence does not have to lead to an addiction, at least not one that is easy to spot. Some sufferers from codependence let their job, their success, or the accumulation of wealth become their main source of self-confidence. People of this kind will often appear extremely successful and driven, yet they are internally plagued with a never-ending need for increased material worth in order to feel a sense of self. In a person such as this a job loss or even retirement can cause severe depression, since his supply of self-worth has suddenly run dry. Others derive their identity from a role they play in society or family. A parent may achieve his or her sole sense of being from the children and their successes. Some use their relationship with others, as spouses, lovers, or just friends, as their wellspring of identity. Whenever the source of validation is sought in another person, one form of relationship addiction or another is liable to develop.

One thing to remember is that the unifying characteristic of any form of codependence is the need for an outside form of self-validation. This can lead to a number of different behaviors or roles a person will play in order to receive the desired feedback. Some people will act meek and accommodating in order to gain the approval of the people they depend upon. Others will take on a more aggressive role and become domineering and controlling, seeking their sense of worth in the lives they influence. But controlling behavior does not have to be malicious in intent. Many a codependent will be the epitome of helpfulness to others, but will become emotionally destitute when opportunities for helping others are not available. In this case the codependent derives self-worth from being of service. Again, all these variations have one thing in common - the goal is for the codependent to gain the external feedback required to feel like a worthwhile person. The difference in how this need is placated or what "role" the codependent person engages in leads to the varying diagnoses we encounter in professional literature. The narcissist, the social dependent, both act out their differing personality traits from similar codependent roots.

To confuse us even more, a single codependency sufferer may not be limited to only one of the possible behaviors. Some codependents engage in both submissive and dominant roles depending on the person they are with and the situation in which they find themselves. When trying to determine whether we suffer from one form of codependence or another it is important to remember that these diagnoses are merely guidelines. They are not absolute or mutually exclusive categories. Plus, when trying to self-diagnose or even through a professional diagnosis we can fall into the trap of labeling ourselves or others. One should never forget that every person is an individual, with individual needs, traits, and inherent worth. Diagnosis is a tool for understanding and should not be used to put limits on people's ability to grow and learn. We may suffer from codependent traits, but they do *not* define who we are and what we are worth.

How do addictions play into this? An "addiction" is a repetitive behavior a person engages in to placate a deep-rooted need, to gain some sort of "high," or lessen the impact of a perceived physical or emotional pain. Since codependence is most definitely a deep-rooted need it is easy to see how it can connect to an addiction. The hallmark of a true addiction is that the addict, apart from initial short-term gratification, encourages long-term damages to body, mind, social and/or material standing. Oftentimes an addict will become aware of the detriment of his or her addictive behaviors but will feel unable to stop. The addict feels that life and normal functioning are not possible without engaging in the addiction. Over time, the addiction becomes the most important factor in the addict's life. Most of his or her mental and emotional focus centers on whatever form the addiction takes. Drug addicts feel as if they exist only to acquire more drugs. A love addict's only obsession will be the relationship he or she cherishes above all else. As the addiction progresses, an addict tends to sacrifice more and more of his or her life, interests, resources, and sense of self to it. Over time it often feels as if the addiction has taken over every part of life. These trends appear common to almost all forms of addictive behavior, regardless of the addiction's focus. Since almost any outside source can become the fuel for an addiction, even such things as plastic surgery or dieting, it is easy to understand how codependency can cause so many different and dangerous behaviors. Yet in the end, whatever the addiction may be, it does not give the sufferer what he wants. After all, no outside source will manage to truly fill the emotional hole a codependent individual wishes to fill.

Another hallmark of addiction is that once an addict has engaged in the drug of choice, he or she will feel a short period of satisfaction, elation, and euphoria. In drug use and alcoholism this is achieved by the high or buzz received from the imbibed substance. Gamblers are known to experience a thrill during high-stakes betting, a sex addict may only live for his sensual gratification. Even a love addict tends to feel euphoric when a new relationship has begun. Everything is fresh, everything is new, and hope is boundless. Yet, like all true addictions, this "high" phase is inadvertently followed by the equivalent of a hangover or going "cold turkey." When the relationship breaks up or the love addict realizes that despite being in a relationship he still does not feel fulfilled the "crash and burn" occur. What follows this "low" phase is that the addict will seek out more of his/her personal drug of choice.

An alcoholic will return to drinking, a love addict will seek a new and better lover; a more "perfect" person to love. Popular Twelve-Step programs for various forms of addiction define "insanity" as "engaging in the same behavior over and over again and expecting different results." One has to realize that many addicts will, at one point or another, come to realize the futility of their actions. Some will even desire to be freed of their addiction and attempt to abstain from it for a while. Oftentimes these attempts fail. How often have we heard from people who tried to quit gambling or drinking and went back to their old habits? How many people with serial relationships swore off them only to start the same pattern over again? And even if a codependent manages to let go of an addiction, a new one may very well take its place.

All of this may sound depressing and hopeless. Anyone reading this and recognizing their own behaviors might very well feel their situation is also hopeless. I can assure you this is not the case. As frightening as these issues may be, they are far from insurmountable. But in order to heal, we must first learn to understand what it is we need to address. By understanding the differences between addictive behaviors and the codependent attitudes at their root, we can begin to not only curb engaging in the addiction, but to undo the beliefs and motivations that fostered them. Codependence is something that is learned over time, by our upbringing and social conditioning. Addictions can be the means codependents use in an attempt to alleviate the pain of their inner emptiness. Yet almost all attempts to fill an internal, emotional void through external measure fail over time. The means to fill this "hole of the soul" is better found in self-discovery and self-love. All the successful programs, books, and therapies that deal with codependence have one thing in common: they focus on letting people find their own, innermost source of worth and confidence. A diagnosis of codependence or addiction is not the end, nor is it a death sentence. It is an opportunity to finally become whole.

Chapter 2: A "Good" Childhood

A lot of people think a 'bad' childhood is what causes addiction problems. They assume the parents of individuals who suffer with addiction were (or are) alcoholics, drug users, or child abusers. It's true for some of these people. In fact, it's probably true for a lot of them. But those who suffer with codependency and relationship addiction can also have 'good' childhoods, in that their parents were there for them and nurtured them. Excessively. While this might seem wonderful when it's taking place, it's actually doing the child a great disservice. Children who are closely sheltered by their parents, and children who have everything done for them all the time, generally don't learn to do things for themselves or be independent human beings, either physically or emotionally. In many cases they grow up lost, confused, and easily frightened when exposed to the world around them. In short, they learn to depend on others for even their basic needs, because they've never been forced to do anything for themselves. This was my childhood.

My parents did *everything* for me, and even now, as I work my way from my late thirties into my early forties, they still often try to 'help' me in the form of controlling what I do. They offer suggestions, but you can tell pretty easily that they think theirs is the suggestion I should take. They never say 'I told you so,' but you can see it in their eyes when I refuse one of their suggestions and make a choice that doesn't turn out well for me – and there's really no guarantee their suggestion would have turned out any better. I know they mean well, and they only want to help. I'm at fault as well, for letting them do this for so long. I lived to please them. I felt I was not worthy of their attention, and in my desperate attempt to feel that worth, I allowed them to completely control me. I craved their approval, and I felt I had to have it or I wouldn't be worth anything. After all, how good a person could I be if I was a disappointment to my parents?

Often, when you hear sad stories of codependency and addiction problems, it's because parents didn't take the time to be with their children – to be present in their lives and teach them right from wrong. You hear stories of abuse and neglect, and I am in no way trying to make light of these stories. They are tragic, and painful, and I wish for all the world they didn't have to happen. These children were forced through circumstances beyond their control to learn things the hard way, and many of them develop lifelong problems that could have been avoided. What most people never see, though, is the other side of the coin. Living an excessively sheltered life can be just as detrimental to a child as being allowed to live too freely. When you keep your children too close to you, both physically and emotionally, they don't have the opportunity to develop their own humanity. Most people can't see that. How could having loving parents possibly have been a *bad* thing?

The fact that I wasn't able to function on my own was something I only realized gradually. It wasn't something I thought about much when I was little. As a kid, who wants to do chores and learn to cook and clean and stuff anyway? I thought never having to do any of that made me privileged. After all, I got an allowance – and a pretty healthy one – for doing amazingly little work. There was no way I was going to volunteer for more. That might sound like a lot of laziness, but you were a kid once. Remember how much you didn't want to do? You wanted to do only what *you* wanted to do, which is pretty selfish, but that's the way children are. They aren't selfish in a malicious way, usually. They're just selfish because they haven't yet developed enough to 'know better' and understand why and how helping others can also benefit them. And they don't think about later, when they might *need* to be able to cook and clean and do the laundry. Many of them can't balance a checkbook or shop for groceries, and even older children and teenagers often can't do these things. I know I couldn't do those things as a teenager, but I probably should have been able to.

My mother was still doing my laundry, cleaning my room, and fixing my lunches when I was seventeen years old. Part of the reason behind it was that I wasn't going to do it if I didn't have to. That was my fault. The other part of it was that my mother never asked me to do anything, and simply did it all herself. That was her fault. But maybe 'fault' isn't even a fair term. I didn't know any better. She didn't know any better. That mostly absolves us of our guilt. We simply were not aware of the dangers we were causing for ourselves and other people later down the line. Everyone tries to raise their children the best way they can, if they are conscientious and caring parents, and my parents' goal was to make my life as comfortable and easy as possible, as long as it was done on their terms. Because they tried so hard to do that they actually made it harder for me, especially as I got older, but I don't fault or blame them. Their intentions were good and honorable, even if I didn't turn out quite the way they'd hoped.

Most people might think my mom would be the most possessive and controlling because she was the one who ran the household while my father was at work, but she wasn't. My father was right there with her. In my later teenage years, if I had a date dad waited up for me, just to make sure I got home safely (at an early curfew, of course). I remember once, at sixteen years old, I had a midnight curfew. I wasn't even on a date. I was out with a female friend. We had been at the beach and lost track of time and it wasn't like today, with technology all over the place. I didn't have a cell phone or any other way to contact my parents. I drove like a madwoman, but I was five minutes late getting home, and my father was pacing back and forth, back and forth, in the front yard. And he insisted to me in later years that he never worries about anything. Sure.

That wasn't the first time he acted that way, and it wasn't the last, either. Overprotective was a massive understatement. It's possible to love and protect someone too much, and the results can be disastrous. Some kids rebel to a harsh extent, involving themselves with drugs and alcohol and dangerous practices like unprotected sex. I didn't do any of those things, which is good, but I just held all the worries and problems and feelings of being trapped inside, which is bad. I felt smothered much of my life, and yet I was afraid to move away from that smothering influence because it was all I knew. It's amazing what a person can get used to, and what they learn to tolerate as being 'normal.' Don't get me wrong. I love my parents very much, and they are truly good people at heart. They just loved me too much when I was a child, and they still do. But I'm getting ahead of myself.

Some of my very earliest childhood memories – from when I was four or five years old – are of lying in bed between my parents. It's after the 10:00 o'clock news, and everyone has just settled in. I never had a 'bedtime' when I was little. I went to bed when my parents went to bed. Sometimes I fell asleep earlier, and I remember my father carrying me, but not usually. I was tucked in between mom and dad, curled on my side, and I slept there, making sure my ear was covered up so nothing would get it while I slept. I was so phobic about that ear - and other things, too. For a while I didn't sleep…I only lay awake, scared to close my eyes. I thought if I fell asleep I might die, but if I stayed awake I'd be OK. It was the first signs of an anxiety disorder that still occasionally plagues me today, over thirty years later, but I didn't know it back then. I thought everyone lay awake at night, fearing death. I thought it was normal. It wasn't until my actual panic attacks started in my early twenties that I was able to look back and realize that I'd always been anxious. I firmly believe that anxiety is part of what contributed to my relationship problems, codependency, and depression – problems that will always be with me and I can only learn to control, not do away with.

I never even had my own bedroom, or my own bed, until I was ten years old. Most people would be appalled by that today. I wouldn't be surprised if someone reading this draws the conclusion that something was 'going on' between my parents and myself because I slept in their bed for so long and was so close to them. There are a lot of stories that sound similar and then later the adult child provides shocking revelations that her mother or father (or both) molested her when she was little, and she just remembered it, after all those years. I do understand how those kinds of things can happen, and I also understand how people can 'forget' those kinds of things for many years. The human mind does *not* want to remember those sorts of things, and it can block them out until something in later life triggers them for some reason. Let me assure you that was not the case with my parents and me, ever. I was fortunate to never be put in the position where the parental love that my mother and father lavished on me turned into something else. I am not in any kind of denial, and I have no repressed memories. My parents were codependents, not child molesters.

I slept my childhood nights away, tucked between my parents, and I still didn't feel safe. On weekend mornings, when I didn't have to get up for school, mom got up early but I would lie in bed next to my dad, and eventually I would wake him up so I wouldn't have to be alone. I was too afraid to get up by myself and go up the long hallway to the kitchen. Wait, now. Really *read* what I just said there. I was *too afraid,* in my own house, where I had lived since I was a baby, to be alone for the length of time it took for me to climb from a bed, cross a room, and walk (or run) up a hallway to where my mother was. I was that anxious, and that dependent, because with the exception of school I was never away from at least one of my parents. Ever. How sad, now that I look back on it, but of course I didn't see it then. You don't, when you're a kid. Even as an adult, you often don't see the problems you have. You're too close to them, and it takes someone else to point them out to you – or sometimes time has a way of doing it for you, as you get older.

At the time, though, I just thought I was enjoying a wonderful, close relationship with my parents, and I thought everyone had fear like that – fear of 'things' coming out of the woodwork to get you, fear of dying, fear of being alone. I didn't realize I had an anxiety disorder – those kinds of things weren't talked about back then, and not as much was even known about them. I didn't realize that my parents were codependent, and that they were raising me to be that way as well. Who would think of that, as a kid? And back in the 1970s codependency and other addictions weren't talked about like they are now. Instead, they were just swept under the rug. Most people (like my parents) didn't know these mental and emotional issues existed and if they *had* known, they wouldn't have believed they were real, or that they could be a problem for them or for those they loved.

For children today, things are a little different. Mental health issues are more understood, and people are more accepting of the idea that mental health issues don't make a person 'crazy.' Not everyone understands codependency or relationship addiction, though, and many who acknowledge the reality of these conditions just want a pill they can take to 'fix' them. There isn't a pill for those particular problems specifically, but even if there was, I'm not convinced it would be the best choice. Masking the symptoms doesn't get to the root of the problem, where real work to correct and control it can begin. For the people who are adults now, especially those who are middle-aged or older, the old ideas that mental health conditions aren't 'real' often still prevail. That hurts the people who need help, and it hurts the friends and family members of these people. If you're in that 'it's not real' group, please understand that it *is* real, and that you could be living a much happier life if you'd be willing to open yourself up to the possibilities and the help that's out there.

One of my biggest hurdles was that my father came from the 'my word is law' generation, which you might be familiar with if you're in your late thirties or older. He also had a lot of interest in the 'I haven't heard of that and/or don't understand that, so it must not be true' school of thought. Anyone else have a parent like that? I think they're pretty common, really. My father was forty years old before I was born. I was the only child of a marriage that has lasted more than fifty years and is still going strong. I've been told that I'm very rare as I approach my fortieth year of life, because my parents are both still living and still married to one another.

It's unusual, today, but back when they got married you just didn't get divorced. People stayed together, and they overlooked things. I don't know that their marriage is unhappy...I think by now it's mostly just a comfortable habit. They still occasionally flirt with each other, and it always makes me smile to see that, or to see the impish grin that my father gets...I can imagine what he must have looked like when he was young and strong and my mother fell in love with him. My father was the provider, and my mother was the homemaker, and now they are both retired and can do what they want. I don't really think they know what that is, though, and I hope they find out before it's too late.

My mother came from the 'listen to your man' generation, and the 'just store up the anger/pain/disappointment and don't say anything' school of thought. She rarely spoke her mind to my father, and I never saw them fight when I was little. Even today, I don't see them quarrel. Mom says something, dad says 'yes' or 'no,' and that's the end of it. His word is law.

Part of my 'problem' was that I grew up on seventy-five acres in the desert southwest. We didn't even have a street address. We had a post office box in town where we got our mail and a washed-out section of road that would flood and race like a river if it rained too hard, stopping us from getting to town if we were home and getting home if we were in town. My parents and relatives got vehicles stuck there once or twice, as well. At night, there were no security lights and no street lights. Sometimes, my father and I would take a flashlight and a blanket out to the bed of his pickup truck, and we would lie there and look at the stars and talk about whether there was life out there. Was it like us? Was it looking back? Were we a noticeable point of light in someone or something else's night sky? We would talk about those questions and others while night creatures made noise around us and coyotes howled in the distance. Sometimes, dad and I would sit around a campfire in our front yard and roast marshmallows and talk about the same kinds of questions.

It looked like the setting for every Western movie ever made. My backyard was a mountain, my gray-stucco home nestled in the abandoned crater of an old volcano, my aunt's home, in that same crater, was rumored to have been built on an old Indian burial ground. I don't know if that was really true, but I know I heard and saw some strange things there. I can't explain them but I know they were real, and I wasn't the only one. I wasn't interested in spirituality then, so I had no interest in such things, other than to be afraid of them. I wasn't even particularly religious. My parents did not attend church, but they did believe in God. They told me about Him, and about Jesus, in a half-hearted and round-about way, and they pretty much left the rest of it alone. I had no other kids around to play with or ask questions of. All I knew were my parents, and a couple of other adult relatives who lived close – my aunt, two uncles, and a cousin who was much older than I was. Later on I developed a few friendships, but for most of my formative years it was just me and my parents in our scenic Western wonderland.

I struggled in school, but not with the academic side of things. I did very well in all my work, earning high marks and not forgetting to do my homework. I turned things in on time, I didn't miss a day of school, and I didn't talk in class or disrupt anything, all in a desperate attempt to gain acceptance and love – to forge relationships. For that, I was ridiculed. My Kindergarten teacher called my mother in for a conference, wanting me to repeat my Kindergarten year because I didn't play with the other children or interact in the way that the teacher thought I should. The school thought I might be handicapped or slow, despite my high grades. My mother was nice the first time, but after she was called in a second time for the same thing she wasn't as polite. Have you ever seen a female tiger? Beautiful and sleek, and seemingly unconcerned about others nearby. Just try to bother her cub, though, and she'll tear your head off. That was my mom. The teacher never called her in again, and I went on to first grade with the rest of my class.

In truth, it wouldn't have mattered had I repeated Kindergarten. It wouldn't have changed who I was. I wasn't comfortable with anyone but my parents and the people I knew in my immediate family. I knew only how to interact with them and how to act like an adult. I was intelligent and serious and not particularly athletic or attractive. My sense of humor was dry and sarcastic. I was basically misunderstood by my peers. I didn't want to play with kids my age. They played 'baby games' and were stupid, in my opinion. Ever heard the term 'too smart for your own good'? It's really possible. I wouldn't trade my high intelligence for anything today, but I can't say it made my life any easier when I was young. Other children don't like someone who's smarter than they are, and the smart child doesn't like to play with others who can't interact at his or her intellectual level. I was overly shy and backward up until my senior year of high school, when I slowly began to branch out. Unfortunately, getting to know more people set me up for more relationships, which set me up for more problems. Maybe it would have been better if I would've just continued to keep to myself, but I'll never know. We have to play the hand we're dealt.

From first grade on through my eleventh grade year (after which I moved across the country and no one at school knew who I was) I was a target for a lot of other children. Gangs of popular girls would tease me, kids would stick the ever-popular 'kick me' signs on the back of my jacket, boys would laugh at me and joke about my underdeveloped chest, asking if I was a boy or a girl, because they couldn't tell. My short, frizzy hair didn't help, and my parents shopped for my school clothes at discount stores that never carried anything fashionable. I don't know whether I'll ever get over that lingering feeling that someone is out to find a way to make fun of me. If you walk up to me today and pat me on the back, it won't be long before you'll see me surreptitiously checking to make sure you didn't stick some kind of rude sign on me while you were patting. I know it's silly. Adults generally don't play those kinds of cruel jokes. But I still check. When you hear people say 'that scarred me for life,' that's the kind of thing they're talking about.

As I got older, the emotional taunting got worse. Anything a person could be picked on for, I was picked on for. I don't intend to make this into a 'poor me' sob story, but I think it's important to have an understanding of what I went through, and how I felt about it. The way I was treated by others contrasted so strongly with the way I was treated by my parents that it created moments of great conflict and existential angst, and it ultimately shaped who I became in my teens and twenties, and even into my early thirties. There was no way for a young mind to reconcile the idea of parental love with the idea of perceived societal hate. I realize now that it wasn't that society hated me. The children who teased me probably didn't even really hate me. They just knew I was different, so they made fun of me. It's just what children do. If I'd been like them, I would've been accepted and probably no one would've bothered me. I used to hate being different. Now I love it. It's all a matter of time and perspective.

When I was around ten, and finally moved into my own bedroom, I developed a couple of friendships – but they weren't really friendships in the truest sense. They were more along pity-friendship lines, and I was the one being pitied. One of the first 'friends' I developed was a distant relative. She was only a couple of years younger than me, and she was raised in a different kind of dysfunctional household than mine. In her home, dad hit and yelled at mom for burning the roast at dinner, and then we got to listen to the springs squeak later that night as they 'made up.' That was the life she grew up in. Despite this she managed to get married only once and stay that way, have several children, and establish a good career. Is she happy, really? I have no idea. I never talk to her, and only find out anything about her through other relatives' occasional comments. No one in my extended family talks to me or my parents much. I guess they're all too busy with their own lives. Even those who we were close to when I was young basically shunned us after we moved away to another state. It seems to be a sin in my family to do something 'out of the norm.'

I couldn't really figure out what was wrong with me that no one seemed to want my friendship. I shared my lunches, my toys, my ideas, and my homework. I did everything for the person who I was 'friends' with, or who I wanted to be friends with, but it never, ever seemed to be enough. In hindsight, I think I tried *too* hard. I would be willing to bet that other kids could almost smell the desperation on me when I tried to be their friend. Some of them ignored me and some of them used me, but it ended up the same when all was said and done. My parents tried to help by providing me with clichés, such as the tried-and-true 'if they don't want to be friends with you, it's their loss.' They also told me to ignore the teasing and all kinds of other things, but they never actually *did* anything – and neither did I. I didn't know what to do. I worshipped my parents. If what they told me to do wasn't working, how could there be anything else that would? Was it possible that they really didn't know how to fix my problem? That was an incredibly scary thought.

I couldn't understand how my parents could not know something. I believed my parents – especially my dad – literally knew everything and could solve any and every problem, no matter what it dealt with. The idea that I was relying on people who might not be reliable was frightening and confusing. Today, I would know how to deal with that, but as a kid I was at a complete loss. I didn't even know who I could talk to about it. I didn't know anyone else *to* talk to. So I just kept my mouth shut and suffered. I tried to act happy at home so my parents would be happy, because I wanted so much to please them. If telling them about my problems at school didn't change anything, it would be useless to keep telling them the same things over and over again. I did my crying in private as often as I was able. At school I kept silent, kept my head down, and tried to go unnoticed. I avoided the other kids when I could, and tried to stay near teachers and others who could intervene if trouble got started when avoidance wasn't possible. It didn't always work, but it probably saved me from even further abuse at the hands of other children who had no concept of (or concern for) how much pain they were causing me.

While the pain of the teasing was bad, the conflict between loving my parents and not understanding why they weren't giving me a magic answer to fix my problems at school was much worse. If they couldn't solve my problem, it was possible that there were other things they didn't know, or were wrong about. But there was another, far worse, possibility. Maybe they really didn't love me as much as they said they did. Maybe it was just that they were stuck with me as their child and were trying to pretend they cared. Maybe they were just trying to make the best of a bad situation. That thought terrified me. It kept me from sleeping, and I tried to please them more and more. I usually did everything they said, without question, and the few times I did rebel I felt horrible for it. I sobbed and clung to them and literally begged for forgiveness, no matter how slight the infraction. Even though they always said it was OK, I was never really convinced in my mind and in my heart that it was – and it was through no actual fault of theirs. They never once honestly acted as though they didn't care about me. I was just that afraid of losing the only security I knew.

I was clearly addicted to my parents, even though I was conflicted about whether they really loved me. I felt guilty even thinking that they might not have all the answers and might not care enough to really give them to me if they did, but it was something that wouldn't leave my mind. I dreaded going to school, where I knew the harassment would continue. I know almost all kids get teased about something or other during their school careers, but the kind of pain I was subjected to went above and beyond what most people have to endure. We had one boy in our school who never bathed and wore the same clothes to school every day. He never brushed his hair or his teeth, he smelled terrible, and he wasn't very smart. He was teased less than I was.

I'm not sure what it was about me that people found to be such a target for their harassment. I wasn't good at sports, and I was shy and naïve, but I don't think that was it. I don't even think it was getting branded 'teacher's pet' at an early age because

I was smart and didn't talk in class or cause trouble. I think it was just because I was different – and the crooked teeth, coke-bottle glasses, and home-permed hair gone wrong didn't really help anything, either. I was also told by the school nurse that I had scoliosis, which is an abnormal curvature of the spine, and a heart murmur caused by a mildly-prolapsed mitral valve, but my parents shrugged these things off. I never went to the doctor for either one of them, or for anything else.

I don't think my parents were capable of understanding that there might actually be something wrong with their precious baby girl – or maybe they really didn't care about me, and they didn't want to waste their money on things like visits to doctors. They treated me like I was perfect, though, no matter what I did or said. I'll bet a lot of people wish their parents thought they were so perfect that they never got into trouble for anything. If you're one of them, you really shouldn't be jealous. I promise it wasn't everything you'd think. Instead of enjoying the fact that I could get away with murder, I spent my childhood – and most of my adult life – agonizing about the fact that I *knew* in my heart I wasn't good enough for all that praise, and I wasn't at all worthy of the kindness and love I was receiving from my parents. It didn't take long for me to start feeling like I was a bad person, and I was just hiding it so well that my parents hadn't caught on yet. When they did, I thought they would stop loving me for sure, and then I really *would* be all alone.

As I got into my later childhood and teenage years, the pattern I had with female friends when I was younger began to show up in relationships with boyfriends. I had a lot of crushes on boys who wanted nothing to do with me, and the few boys I did date were not popular, attractive, or well-liked by others. They were outcasts, like me. I don't know what happened to any of them. I never bothered to keep in touch. I can only hope they grew up to finally escape their outcast status, and that they are happy now, wherever they are. Sometimes I think of them, and I wonder if any of them remember me. I suppose it doesn't really matter, but that need to be accepted and understood that I felt so strongly in childhood still sometimes shows up, and when it does I want to be remembered fondly, even if it's only by someone I knew for a brief period of time twenty or twenty-five years ago.

Most people could care less, but those of us with relationship addiction worry about those kinds of things, even if we try to ignore them and pretend they don't matter.

When things didn't work out with a boy, I found the same kinds of excuses for those relationships as I used for friendships that ended with other girls. He wasn't nice, or he isn't smart, or all kinds of other things. The truth was, though, that it was usually me who ended the relationship…and it was usually because I didn't really want to go out with that particular boy in the first place. I usually had my heart set on some great-looking guy who played a lot of sports and didn't do very well in his studies and had absolutely *no clue* that I existed. I wanted what I couldn't have, always. The boy who was totally unavailable to me. Remember the torch bearer from Chapter One? I carried a torch for the boy I could never get. He was usually very popular, and so was his cheerleader girlfriend. I had to know where he lived, and I had to find his phone number – even though I would never, ever call it. Sometimes I had a class with that boy, and I wouldn't do as well in that class, because I was daydreaming. Everybody gets crushes, but this was torch bearing, bordering on obsession. Very, very unhealthy.

During the time all of this was going on, I was also a saboteur. I usually had a boyfriend, but he wasn't popular or particularly attractive. He was the kid who had a lot of acne and was too fat or too skinny and played the trombone or the tuba in the band. He was probably in the chess club or some other club populated by kids that the 'in crowd' judged to be geeks and/or nerds of the highest order. He was probably a perfectly nice boy, too, and he probably wanted people to care about him and value him just as much as I wanted people to care about and value me. Most of the boys who played in the band or were in the chess club or were otherwise considered nerdy were nice, even if they weren't the kind of physical specimen most girls want.

But I found a reason to wreck the relationship, because he wasn't who I really wanted. And I was angry…angry at the thoughts that kept running through my head, saying that I didn't deserve anyone who I thought was 'better.' Why in the world did I think that guy was better, anyway? I was rejecting perfectly nice people to pursue the kind of people society said were worthwhile, and not giving any thought to the quality of the person on the inside, only what he looked like. Who was I, that a good-looking guy might notice me? I was ugly, even if my parents said I was beautiful.

I knew better, and I added that knowledge onto the idea that there were some discrepancies between what my parents said and what I saw on the news, read in books or magazines, or heard from others. I tried to ignore this, because it helped to enforce the idea that my parents really didn't know everything. They kept saying what a wonderful person I was, but all evidence at school indicated otherwise, unless you counted my grades and some of the teachers who seemed to like me simply because I didn't cause them a problem. I often felt that they were nice to me out of pity. They felt sorry for me. Not everything my parents said matched what I discovered to be true through 'book-learning.' And my father had some prejudiced tendencies I hadn't found to be accurate in the real world. I wasn't sure whether to believe the evidence of my own eyes, or decide that I must be disillusioned and simply believe everything my parents said as the gospel truth. See how confused I was? I was actually contemplating *ignoring the real world* in favor of my parents' beliefs, just like I did when I was very, very young.

For a while, that's almost what I did. As I got into high school I held some of my own opinions, but I kept them to myself. I agreed with my parents out loud, even if I didn't agree with them on the inside. For example, I didn't say anything to my father when he saw a criminal on the nightly news and used…well, the 'n-word.' I don't say it, and I won't say it here. I think it's offensive, despite the fact that I grew up in a family and a society where it was used quite frequently. In my father's defense, however, I think it's just the way he was raised (and I don't mean that makes it OK, it just helps to indicate a reason). He has a few black friends, and he likes them, and he treats them well. He never calls them 'that word.' In his father's generation, that was what you called *all* black people. In his generation, that was what you called *bad* black people. In my generation, at least in my opinion, that is what you *don't* call black people. Whether you're a good person and a valuable member of society has nothing to do with the color of your skin or where you come from. But I digress.

My father and mother held then, and hold now, a lot of opinions I don't share, but no one's going to agree on everything. We could've argued for days on the death penalty, politics, religion, and countless other topics, but back then I wasn't willing to risk ruffling feathers, and now I know I'm much happier if I just agree to disagree and get on with my life. As a kid, though, and even as a teenager, the feather-ruffling was the biggest concern for me, and the biggest reason I kept my mouth shut. How would they react if they knew I didn't think exactly like they did? I just didn't know.

I had no self esteem and no confidence in any of my abilities. Everything that was 'me' came from my relationship to my parents, or so I thought at the time. Because I had grown up so dependent on them, I looked to them for every answer. I didn't know how to do anything, but most importantly I didn't know how to think for myself. The thoughts and ideas I had that didn't match those of my parents? Well, they must be wrong. Why would I be taught something by people who professed to love me if it wasn't true? But how could they be right all the time? I went back and forth on the issue for most of my teenage years. Part of me wanted to simply rebel and run away, leaving no forwarding address. The bigger part of me insisted how incredibly stupid I was being by thinking that way. After all, I didn't know how to do anything, remember? I'd never even had a job, and I'd spent all of my allowance money. How was I supposed to make it? And would they hate me if I left? Could they live without me? I didn't know the answers to those questions, either. So I stayed, and was assimilated.

Around that same time, I acquired my first serious boyfriend, which was my first real foray into unhealthy and codependent relationships that didn't involve family members. When I first met Steven[1] I was fourteen and he was sixteen. I

---

[1] All names of friends/boyfriends/husbands/family members, both past and present, as well as all identifying characteristics and all state/city names have been changed to protect privacy.

thought he was cool, because he had a car...sort of. Oh, it was four wheels and a motor, but that was about all you could say about it. It was a lime green contraption with many dents in it, I don't recall him ever washing it, and the gas pedal stuck. I remember him cruising by the high school one morning and waving to me from the passenger seat. There was no one driving, but that stuck pedal just propelled the car right on by. I thought he was an idiot, but in a good and funny way. He was a kind-hearted soul with a lot of problems. That started my relationship pattern early. I felt I could rescue him – from what I'm not really sure...from himself, I suppose. His home life was terrible, at least from what he said about it during numerous conversations, and although we dated for almost a year, I don't think I ever met his mom and dad or went to his house. He always came to my house or met me somewhere. I guess he could have been leading a secret double life, and I never would have been aware of it. Unlikely, but not impossible.

Eventually he moved away, and that effectively ended our relationship. Oh, we tried to stay in touch, but long-distance romances rarely work, especially between teenagers. Eventually, we just stopped writing, and email wasn't around then. People had to write an actual letter and mail it and wait patiently to get one back. I missed him incredibly, though. I had been with him for what seemed like a very long time, and he had said he wanted to marry me when we got older. I actually believed him, and I wanted to be married. I felt it would make my life complete because I would have someone who I could learn to take care of, and that would make my parents proud of me. When Steven moved away, it was hard to just forget that and let it go. Rather than wait for him, though, I had to have a relationship. I didn't know how to be without one. I was so used to being so close to my parents, and I was used to being close to Steven. I needed closeness again, so I could be happy. So I embarked on a series of relationships, looking for 'the one.'

I dated a geeky, scrawny guy from the school band for about ten minutes, and then I started dating a Latino boy who was four years older than me. He was a senior and I was only a freshman, and my father was *very* angry. The age difference was a problem for him, and so was the racial difference. This boy was 'not like us,' and therefore unacceptable. Plus I think he worried that, with the age difference, the boy would want much more in the way of a physical relationship than I needed to be involved with. I didn't really like the boy that much anyway, so I broke up with him. It made my dad happy, so I felt like he wouldn't turn his back on me for doing something he didn't agree with. He used to say he was very disappointed in me when I did something he didn't like. I don't think he ever understood how much that hurt. He never hit me, but I think it would have been less painful than knowing I was a disappointment to him. I didn't really have the concept of what he meant when he said that.

You see, I couldn't put it in perspective back then. My thought was that, if my father said he was disappointed in me, he was really disappointed in *me* – all of me. My life, therefore, was a disappointment to him. It made me feel like I was completely worthless, and I was constantly worried about being a disappointment to him and to my mother. I think I was worried more about my father though, since I was pretty much a 'daddy's girl' when I was young. When he expressed his disappointment with me, I worried that he was disappointed that I existed at all. Time has shown me this was not the case. He was only disappointed in the choice I made at the time, but it's taken me years to figure that out. Even as I write these words today, more than twenty years later, I worry about my father's opinion of me and I crave his approval, even though I understand the unhealthiness of that and continue to work on it. It is not something I can change overnight and I accept that, difficult as it might sometimes be.

The only thing in my childhood that caused me to be rebellious to any noticeable degree was a relationship I developed with another girl. She was the same age as I was, she was a rebel, she was a lesbian, and she was beautiful. We were both sixteen years old. I had lived with such a sheltered upbringing that I didn't know she was a lesbian. I didn't even know what a lesbian *was* when I first met her. I thought she was just friendly. She seemed like the first friend I had ever made who genuinely *liked* me, and she didn't disappear when other kids teased me. She was my bodyguard, and she protected me from others who tried to cause me problems. It might seem hard for you to believe that I didn't see what was going on with her or didn't realize her intentions, but when I said I was sheltered as a child, I meant it. I knew virtually nothing about sex, even at sixteen, and had never experienced any form of it.

This new friend, Margaret, wanted to spend all her time with me. My parents didn't like her from the start. I understood later that it was because she was a bad influence on me and into all kinds of trouble-making things she shouldn't be into, but at the time I just thought they wanted to sabotage the one, seemingly true friendship I'd ever had. I couldn't understand why they would do this to me, when they said they loved me and wanted me to be happy. The only time in my life where I actually got in much trouble with my parents was because of Margaret. Although I never became her girlfriend, she did make her intentions clear to me eventually. Naturally, I was curious because I'd never had any kind of interesting experiences. My mild curiosity didn't match that well with her sincere interest in a lifestyle I didn't want. I have nothing against homosexual people, at all. But since I'm not one, the kind of relationship she wanted with me was basically doomed from the start. Add to that the increasing pressure from my parents to stay away from her, and the friendship ended up doomed, as well.

At the time I was very upset about the end of the friendship, but it wasn't so much that I really cared for her as a friend that deeply. There was a lot of drama to our friendship. I was used to the drama, and I craved it. There was always something going on. Some boy liked her, or she was jealous because I liked some boy, or there was something going on at school. It was a fascinating friendship, and there were very few dull moments in it. I longed for that after it was gone. We tried to rekindle our friendship after it ended, but it was unsuccessful. I couldn't hide it from my parents, and she wanted what I was not able to give. She eventually married my male cousin, who was about thirty years her senior, and divorced him after a couple of years. Last I heard, she had found a woman she was very happy with, and they had moved out of state. I wish her well, because I never really believed she meant me any harm.

What my childhood experiences ultimately came down to, and still do come down to under scrutiny, was that I was afraid – both of my parents and of myself. If I challenged my parents, they might not love me anymore. And as I got a little farther into my teenage years a new and even more disturbing thought appeared: If I challenged their beliefs and went my own way, they might think *I* didn't love *them* anymore. They would get old and die, miserable, unloved, and alone. I became convinced I was *that* important to them – that they couldn't live without me. I know now how selfish that was, and how narcissistic for me to think I was the most important thing in their world. They survived for a lot of years before I was born, so they would certainly be all right if I wasn't in their sight twenty-four hours a day, right? Throughout the course of my life, there have been some indications that I might be more important to their happiness than I really should be. They appeared to be just as dependent on me as I was on them. You shall hear about those times, too, as the story goes on.

What I Did Wrong
- Kept my own views to myself even when I knew they were the right ones for me.
- Idolized my parents instead of seeing them as human beings.
- Wasn't willing to speak up when I believed one of my parents was incorrect.
- Pretended to agree with everyone else so as not to make waves or make people not like me – which didn't work, because a lot of people at school didn't like me anyway.
- Didn't insist on help for my anxiety and codependency issues even though I knew something wasn't right.
- Didn't work to explore answers to questions I had about the world – just took my parents' word for it, instead.
- Wasn't willing to learn to do new things and take the initiative in my life, instead of letting my parents do it all for me.
- Didn't insist on getting help with the way I was being treated in school.

What To Look For

- An inability to 'be your own person' because you feel as though people won't accept you.
- Thinking that your parents/siblings/friends won't love you any more if you don't agree with them.
- Thinking that your parents/siblings/friends will feel that *you* don't love *them* if you don't agree with them or try to please them all of the time.
- Deep fear about moving forward or doing anything that might require you to change.
- A need or desire to please others that you can't shake off, even though you may realize it's not healthy.
- Anxiety, panic attacks, or depressive episodes that you don't share with others, or that you share with others but they don't listen to you.
- Being told you're fine, even when you know you're not, just because the people who love you aren't willing to acknowledge you have flaws.
- Constantly seeking acceptance from people even after you've received it from them.

What the Therapist Says

Where in the world does codependence come from? As with so many things in life, there are multiple answers to that. Many people who discover their codependence also realize their childhoods were marked by addictions, alcoholism, or some other sort of dysfunction. Here the word "dysfunction" is used to describe any relationship pattern that becomes unhealthy. Oddly enough, a large number of codependents find that their families of origin never showed any signs of abuse or addiction. Many sufferers of codependence will note that their parents were extremely loving, sometimes overbearingly so. To find the common thread between families where severe abuse and addictions exist and those where loving care is taken to extremes is not apparent at first glance. But when we try to look at the impact both environments can have on a child's self-esteem a common theme emerges.

First, picture a household where one or both parents are severely alcoholic or abuse drugs. Add to this the potential for physical and emotional violence and you get a family environment where a child is faced with a number of painful uncertainties. Anyone who has ever had to deal with a violent alcoholic or addict knows that such a person's behavior is extremely unpredictable. There is no telling what will set such an individual's rage off and cause severe physical and/or emotional harm. Now imagine a child growing up in such a family. This child may never know how to behave in order to avoid harm. Worse, many an attempt by children of violently abusive parents to escape punishment leads to even harsher treatment. Oftentimes the result of an environment such as this is that the child becomes conditioned to believe in his or her own inability to influence life in any form whatsoever. If the parents and/or other family members also engage in emotional abuse, such as telling the child that he or she is utterly worthless, this belief of powerlessness and worthlessness may become the mainstay of the child's self-image. It is easy to see how such a childhood can condition someone to develop codependent traits and low self-worth. The fear of being utterly unable to control one's life or gain love can then give rise to the various behaviors people engage in to cope with codependence. The result is that the cycle of abuse and addiction appears to repeat itself.

But how about a family where the child's needs are catered to in excess? Consider a child who is being showered with love, affection, and all the things she could ever hope for. On the surface such a childhood may appear ideal. Who would not like to be brought up without a care in the world? No chores, no worries, life could be wonderful that way. Yet it is just from such families that a lot of people with codependency issues hail. Once we think about the child's sense of independence fostered in an upbringing of this kind we can start to understand why this would be. After all, how can a child who never has to do anything on his or her own, never has to face uncertainties or tasks without the aid and support of parents, develop a sense of his or her own ability? Also, a child who has never been without the loving support of parents may grow up to feel unable to live without an ever-present loving partner. In a way, this kind of childhood and the abuse environment described previously are direct polar opposites, but can lead to similar forms of codependent patterns. In the first upbringing parents were too emotionally distant and in the second too emotionally enmeshed to allow a child to develop a healthy sense of self-worth and ability.

Of course, many childhoods are not clear-cut cases. Just as with individual diagnoses a person's upbringing can also exhibit a combination of different traits. For example, it is not uncommon for abusive individuals to switch from abuse behavior to overly loving attitudes, what some call the "honeymoon phase." On the same token we have to acknowledge that overly loving relationships can also contain controlling and sometimes abusive behaviors. Abuse and control do not have to be overt, especially when administered verbally. When somebody tells you openly that you are worthless, the resulting lack of self-confidence is easy to spot. But one can instill a belief of being worthless just as well by telling a child that one is only a "good person" when one reaches a certain goal. If that goal is set unreasonably high, maybe even knowingly, and the child has no way to ever achieve it, he may be forced to think he is worthless and "bad." There are many ways that we learn how to think and feel about ourselves. Our parents and family play a huge role in it, but they are not the only source of identity. Our peers, friends, neighbors, the schools and societies we grow up in, they all play their part. Given enough school abuse, even a child from a healthy family can grow up to feel low self-esteem and develop codependence.

Trying to find the reason for one's codependence can be very insightful. To know why we are the way we are can help us in gaining some measure of self-acceptance. But one has to be careful not to use these insights as an excuse for one's own behavior. It would be easy to simply state that since we are the product of our upbringing we are not responsible for what we do. Nothing could be further from the truth. To be able to understand where our innermost beliefs come from is not an excuse, it is an encouragement. Once we learn to understand the mechanisms that create codependence and resulting addictions we can learn the mechanisms to undo them. We also have to acknowledge that oftentimes our parents tried their best to raise us to the best of their ability. Yet just as we can only pass on what we have learned ourselves, they were only able to use the knowledge they had access to. Now that we have new information and learning at our disposal it is our turn to use it to try and better our lives.

One common aspect in people with codependence, especially those with a form of relationship addiction, is an inability to separate their sense of self-worth from their actions. This means that codependents will automatically start feeling bad about themselves when given negative feedback from a person they are emotionally dependent on. If, for example, a loved one disagrees with someone suffering from codependence, that person may feel worthless. The simple act of having the loved one disagree causes the sufferer to feel like he or she is no longer loved. This is an important concept to understand. In some cases the relationship addict may even feel responsible for keeping the partner in a good mood. Of course, this presents the codependent partner with a huge dilemma. There is no possible way he can influence all the factors that might make his partner happy or sad. So, every time a situation comes up where the partner is unhappy this person may feel like a failure. The other person's sadness becomes the relationship addict's responsibility. Codependents with this particular attitude are usually trying to be agreeable to the point where they fear ever voicing an opinion of their own, or even having one.

Another form of this inability of separating an action or another's attitude from one's own sense of self is when the other person's sadness is automatically seen as a personal attack. Codependents who follow these attitudes have difficulty seeing the difference between disagreeing with their opinion and an open attack on them personally. The result can be personal outbursts at any form of criticism. Even though this sort of behavior appears in direct opposition to one who seeks to gain another's approval by always trying to agree, the underlying concept is the same. The person suffering from codependence cannot distinguish between the outside feedback and his or her own sense of self-worth. Faced with such potentially contradictory behaviors it is easy to understand why codependence is such a difficult condition to diagnose. Rather than looking at the behaviors alone, one is forced to determine the motivation behind them in order to understand what is really going on.

Many of the behaviors that people in codependent or addictive relationships engage in put a huge emotional strain on them. Trying to always be agreeable and happy in order to gain someone's approval can be very hard when one is actually not happy at all. In the same way it can be strenuous when we feel we always have to defend our own point of view for fear that disagreement means the other person no longer loves us. In both cases the codependent has to be continuously on guard for fear of the situation changing to a point where the partner no longer gives us positive feedback, which the codependent equates to love and self-worth. In essence, the codependent always feels as though he needs to wear a mask; to play a role in order to be accepted and get the approval he craves. In that manner, the sufferer's already low sense of self-worth is lowered even further. After all, having to wear a mask means that one's own true self is not "good enough." At times a codependent's greatest fear, consciously or subconsciously, can be that other people may see through his masks and discover his true, honest, and totally unlovable self.

The resulting strain can lead to all sorts of stress-related health concerns. Individuals suffering from codependency and resulting addictions are often plagued by various forms of anxiety, depression, bipolar disorder, and sometimes even obsessive-compulsive conditions. Clinical treatment for conditions such as these, medicinal and therapeutic, are now more widely accepted than in previous generations. But the same acceptability has led to a sometimes short-sighted way of dealing with them. Often a person will have anxiety or mood disorders treated without ever considering deeper causes for these maladies. Many times people wind up at a therapist's door, seeking help for a mental condition that ultimately has its root in codependent beliefs. It is with a deeper understanding of the source of such mental conditions that therapy and treatment can be more effective, in both the short and the long term.

Chapter 3: Marriage Number One – Divorced at Eighteen

Ever since I was very young I wanted to be married, and that only intensified after my relationship with Steven ended. I saw teenagers who had gotten married and thought it was a great idea. I watched romantic movies. I smiled at elderly couples who I saw out walking, still holding hands after all those years. I wanted that. I was such a hopeless romantic! Or at least, that's what I thought I was. I still had no clue that I was actually addicted to the idea of the love and romance and happily-ever-after life. When I was in my senior year of high school, there was a girl in my class who had gotten married over the summer, between her junior and senior year. Everyone who met her looked at her stomach. Seeing it was flat, they asked her how old her baby was, or if she had lost the baby. They couldn't understand why in the world she would deliberately get married at that age. She just shrugged it all off. She was in love, and he was in love, and their parents understood, and so they got married. They had no children yet, she was not pregnant, she had not lost a baby or had an abortion, and they were deliriously happy. I knew most people didn't get it, but I did (or thought I did). I believed I understood completely why she did what she did, and I applauded her parents for allowing her to go through with it. Obviously, they believed in her.

Now, in hindsight, I wonder about her. I don't remember her last name, so I can't try to look her up, and I don't know whether she stayed married or not. The same is true of several other former classmates who married their boyfriends either during their senior year or right after. I wish I knew where they were now or how many of them were still married to the same man they married when they were young. Some of them I have tried to find through Internet search engines, but I've not had any luck. Perhaps they've kept a low profile, changed their names, or moved on. I'll probably never know, but I wouldn't be surprised if at least some of them were like me, and got married young for the wrong reasons – the idea of love, the need to be accepted, codependency, a fear of being alone, and other factors.

I was so jealous of people who were engaged or married during my senior year of high school – there was even one girl who got pregnant and married her boyfriend during her junior year – and I just knew I had to get married as soon as possible. What better way to be happy? I would marry young and get an early start, so I could still be spry and coherent at my 50th Anniversary party. I didn't realize at the time why I really had such a desperate need for marriage. Most people don't marry that young. They wait until they're sure they've found the right person. With me, it was more the idea that I had found *a* person, instead of that I had found *the right* person. If someone wanted to marry me I must be valuable and worth something, right? I didn't really stop to consider that the person I was thinking of marrying should be a good person, or it wouldn't help to support my theory that *I* was a good person. So I got married, just over two months after I graduated from high school. I was seventeen years old, and he was nineteen, but in order to understand how we got to that point and why it was such a poor choice, you have to understand how we met and what our courtship was like.

Shortly after Steven and I broke up I dated a series of boys, most of whom I didn't even like very much. It wasn't about liking someone, it was about having a relationship. Someone to call 'mine.' Society expected a 'normal' girl my age to have a boyfriend – and I kept trying to be normal. The more boys I was able to date, however briefly, the more I felt like I was worth something, if all these people liked me. It helped build my self-esteem, but not as much as it would have if these boys had been popular and good-looking. I still felt like I couldn't get boys who fell into that category. When I was just a few months past my fifteenth birthday, I met Daniel. We had a class at school together, even though he was a grade ahead of me.

He was the class clown, always making everybody laugh, and he was a big guy, overweight by probably fifty pounds but still very cute – he carried it well. He, like so many others, decided it would be fun to pick on me, but at least there were fewer things to pick on. I had traded the big, coke-bottle glasses I'd had since fifth grade for contact lenses about the time I started high school, and the frizz the home permanent had given my hair had gone away, leaving me with long, straight brown hair that actually didn't look all that bad. I wasn't really ugly any more, I was just very plain, which was fine by me because I could blend into the background and not be noticed. If I wasn't noticed, I wasn't teased as much.

My teeth still needed braces but my parents insisted they were fine, and my clothes still weren't the most fashionable, but I no longer stuck out so much when placed in a group of my peers. As Daniel continued to tease me, I sensed it was more good-natured than the teasing I had endured from others in the past. The class we were taking together was a photography elective, and Daniel's favorite thing to do was lock us both in the darkroom while our teacher, a kindly older gentleman who didn't deserve to be treated that way, pounded ineffectively on the door and yelled a lot. We never did anything in there, because I was yelling to get out just as loudly as the teacher was yelling to get in. Daniel found it hilarious. His way of showing he liked me was pretty juvenile, really, but I also found it endearing, and on a class trip he finally got the courage, after much harassment by his friends, to ask if he could take me to the prom. Since he was a junior he was eligible to go, and even though I was only a sophomore he could bring anyone he wanted. I accepted, and that prom was our first official date.

I had great hopes for that prom...a beautiful dress, a limousine, all the kinds of things I'd heard other people talking about. I ended up with a thrift-store dress that didn't fit that well, because my parents thought the idea of spending any real money on a dress to be worn only once was just preposterous. They told me how silly it was, and how it was better to be frugal, and how, if Daniel really liked me, he wouldn't care what I wore. And these were people who were making what would have worked out in today's dollars to be a six-figure income. I think mom paid about $40 for my prom dress. There was no limousine. We were allowed to borrow my mother's car so we didn't have to go in Daniel's old pickup truck. Despite all of that, we actually had a really good time. It was awkward at first, with all the romance a prom usually brings and us on our first date. After the prom there was a huge party at the school. I don't remember when my curfew was...I think it was one in the morning. I missed a lot of the all-night party because of that but Daniel called me the next day, and we became a couple in short order, which surprised me.

I didn't think he'd want to continue to spend time with someone like me. Wasn't one evening torture enough?

I had such a pessimistic attitude about myself when I was young. In my eyes I couldn't do anything right. I was ugly, I dressed badly, and I had no personality. We are always our own worst critics. Flaws we see and that seem so glaringly obvious to us are often not even noticed by others unless we take the time to point them out, and who wants to do that? I guess Daniel didn't see my flaws, or if he did he overlooked them, because he seemed very happy with me...for a while. Like any couple, and especially a young couple, we had our problems. We fought for control of the relationship, ourselves, and each other, and no one really seemed to win the battle for very long. Usually I backed down because of my unrelenting fear that I'd be deserted by the people I cared about if I didn't do what they wanted. Unlike my relationship with my parents, I knew Daniel didn't know everything about everything. Rather than believe what he said as the gospel truth I simply agreed with him to avoid trouble. I kept my own opinions – which were still mostly my parents' opinions – to myself.

In the spirit of a lot of young couples we broke up and got back together quite a lot, and there was always drama in our relationship, in our friendships, or both. It seemed like we couldn't go a month without some kind of crisis – either real or perceived – happening in our lives. I wouldn't have known what to do with a healthy relationship if I'd had one, because I was so used to having unhealthy and dependent relationships where drama was the lifeblood of the interactions that took place. One of the main dramatic elements of the relationship that Daniel and I had was courtesy of my friend Margaret. Remember her? Well, even though she liked women, she was still in the process of discovering that and understanding it when we were friends. She still dated boys sometimes, and she seemed to be interested in seeing if she could steal boys from others. One of the boys she wanted to steal was Daniel – presumably just to see if she could. Of course she insisted that wasn't the case, but there were too many things going on that made me suspicious, and they were happening far too often for me to simply ignore them or assume they were coincidental - and that was back when I still believed in coincidence. I don't any more, but that's a story for later.

Of course I had a problem with what she was trying to do, but I had a very difficult time doing anything about it. I didn't want to lose her as a friend because I really didn't make friends very well. On the other hand, I didn't want to lose Daniel because he was the first real boyfriend I'd had since Steven and I had lost touch. They insisted there was nothing going on, and I never actually caught them. Looking back I see an elaborate scheme, but that's only because I know how the rest of the story went.

Our first date was in May, and by October I was convinced I wanted to get married to this man I had only known a few months. I started talking to Margaret about it, and she promised to help me. That worked to further convince me there was nothing going on between the two of them, even though I had been present when he'd shown up at her home late one night with a rose and seemed surprised I was there. He covered it quickly and said she had called him and told him I was there, and he'd come to see me. I wanted to believe that, so I did. Was it realistic? Probably not. I wouldn't fall for that today, but at fifteen or sixteen years old what did I know about the real world? I accepted the explanation because I wasn't willing to challenge anyone, for fear of losing them, and I went on with my life and my plans to get Daniel to marry me. I couldn't just come right out and ask. That would have been too weird, so I left it up to Margaret to find a way.

I don't know what she said or did – and I probably really don't want to know – but Daniel gave me a ring for Christmas. I was thrilled. It was a great ring, I thought. It was a bit too big for me, but I could get that fixed. I wore it home proudly and showed my parents, who pretended to be happy. Later, when I tried to have it sized, I found out it was only gold plated and the stone wasn't real. It wasn't worth anything at all, just a cheap piece of costume jewelry that would turn my finger green if I wore it for very long. I was in shock. I was so angry and so upset, but wait until you hear now naïve I remained. *I thought the jeweler he bought it from had cheated him!*

Hard to believe, isn't it? I look back on it now and wonder how in the world I could have been so incredibly ignorant. I know I'm not stupid, and my MENSA membership has proven that, but ignorance can be available in large amounts, even in the most intelligent of people. It was yet another problem with leading a sheltered life, and another problem with wanting so badly to have a relationship that you will do almost anything and believe whatever is told to you. It's almost like being brainwashed. You do these things just so you don't cause a problem or find out something so terrible that you are forced to end the relationship. You don't think you can live without the person or people you have around you, because you think being whatever you are to them – child, parent, friend, lover, etc. – makes you who you are.

When I confronted Daniel about the ring and told him he'd been cheated, he shrugged it off and said there wouldn't be anything he could do about it now. He convinced me no one would believe him, he couldn't find the receipt, the store wasn't open right then, and countless other excuses. Oh, and he'd spent all his money so he couldn't replace the ring. I wore the fake one until Margaret handed me a note Daniel had written to her, saying he'd only paid twenty dollars for the ring he gave me because he didn't have any money and didn't know if he wanted to get married anyway. Had I had any self-esteem, I would have walked away right then after giving him back the ring and making sure I put it someplace very unpleasant. He shouldn't have lied to me that way – especially not about something so important. That was truly more than a person should have to take from someone who claimed to love her. I was so convinced I would never find anyone else, though, that I tried to stay together with him, despite how hurt I was. It didn't last, and we broke up a few weeks later.

You'd think I would've just moved on, because that's what I had done when Steven and I had broken up, but Steven had moved away, and I saw Daniel every day at school. I missed him, and he seemed to miss me, as well. After some uncomfortable moments for both of us, and a several-week fling I had with a martial arts instructor who was thirty-two years my senior, we got back together, although there was no ring involved, and we managed to do pretty well for a pretty long period of time. We dated all through my junior year – when

Daniel was conveniently a junior again because he had not passed enough of his classes the prior year. We went to homecoming, and we went to prom again, and we spent that night together. It was my first time, and he said it was his, but I doubted that in later years. He seemed to know too much. It didn't really matter, I suppose. What mattered was I thought that had completely convinced him we really should be together always. He did get me a ring after that, a real one although it was tiny and inexpensive, and I wore it for a long time, right up until he asked for it back one cold afternoon, standing on the balcony of his father's house. And then everything changed.

I cried for days and days. I didn't want to give the ring back. Pulling it from my finger was almost more than I could bear, and I begged, literally *begged* him not to take it back from me. Didn't he love me? Didn't all of our time together mean anything? Wasn't I worth it? I guessed not, and he wouldn't really give me straight answers to any of my questions. The rational part of my brain understood why he was doing this – I was moving across the country with my parents. What teenage boy wants to have a long distance relationship? Teenage boys want to cuddle and talk and hug and hold hands and kiss and have sex if they can get it. Other than talking, there isn't much that can be done from 2000 miles away. The rational part of my brain completely understood that, but the rest of my thoughts were in turmoil. The part of me that had spent my entire life needing to belong to someone else was angry, ashamed, and right back into that feeling of worthlessness that I had slowly started to leave by 'belonging' to Daniel. I couldn't find any consolation, anywhere.

Margaret and I had ended our friendship because she continued to spend too much time with Daniel, be too flirty, and try to undermine everything I did. I guess I felt threatened by her, too. With long, wavy hair, bright blue eyes, a deep, sexy voice, full lips, elfish features, large breasts and a tiny waist, she was a threat to almost any other girl – especially one who wasn't too pretty and who was already socially awkward. My parents told me I would find someone new, and someone better than Daniel. They seemed to think this was nothing more than a teenage crush, not love, and it wouldn't matter to me in a few more months. I'd 'get over it' in time, and it wouldn't bother me anymore. I had another friend who I had made at school, but she was little help. She had begun dating the Latino boy I had dated prior to meeting Daniel, and apparently she was so wrapped up in that she really couldn't take or didn't want to take the time to worry about my problems. That left me alone, yet again. Oh, I had people around me, but I was still alone. Have you ever felt alone in a crowd of people? Everyone's laughing and talking and you're right there with them, but you still feel terribly lonely? That was me. I had gotten to the point where I was a bit more accepted – not by the popular kids of course, but I did have several friends. Even with that, loneliness was almost always there, especially when I had to give Daniel his ring back. It was one more reason to feel worthless.

As soon as my junior year was over my parents and I packed up the last of our things, and we traveled across the country from the desert southwest to the Deep South. I went to a new high school for my senior year, and no one knew me there. That was another blow to my already badly-damaged self-confidence, because I suddenly had no friends again. I was back to being totally dependent on my parents for any kind of emotional or mental interaction beyond classroom lectures and learning. I guess I should have looked at it as an opportunity to start afresh and re-invent myself, but I was unable to see that. I didn't see how I might gain anything. All I saw was loss. Loss of friends. Loss of my boyfriend/fiancé. Loss of my self-esteem. Loss of who I was. It was like being set adrift, and the only thing I had to cling to was my parents, so I went right back to doing everything they said and believing everything they believed. It was just easier that way. It felt safe.

Several months later I wrote to Daniel because I couldn't stop thinking about him, and I included my new phone number. He called. Apparently he wasn't as ready to move on as he'd thought he was, because we started talking again. After a few weeks, the wedding was back on. And then it was off. And then it was on. You see the pattern. We broke up and got back together every month or so. He dated other people. I dated other people. Yet we kept hanging on, and we kept coming back to one another. It was incredibly unhealthy. We couldn't seem to make it work, especially long distance, but we couldn't seem to completely let go of one another. Looking back on it now, it was never really love. It was just two people who didn't want to be alone trying to hang on to someone to be there for them, while still trying to look around and see what else was out there. We should have just made a clean break and walked away, but we were both incapable of doing that.

I was torn. I wanted Daniel because we had a history. He had broken my heart asking for his ring back, and now he seemed to want me back. It made me feel valued and worth something. On the other hand, I wanted my freedom. I was in a new state, and I could be someone else now. While I wasn't one of the cool kids, I wasn't teased nearly as much and I'd acquired several friends who were a lot of fun. There were also a couple of boys I really liked, and they were actually aware I existed, so I had hope for something beyond a casual hello in the school hallways. Did I really want to jeopardize all that for someone who had already rejected me more than once? After much debate I decided that I did, and the wedding was back on. He even flew into town to go to my senior prom with me, and my parents allowed him to stay in our home for over a month. We were re-committed to one another when he got on a plane to fly home. A couple weeks later the wedding was off again, and I couldn't even tell you what happened to cause that.

A week later he called me again, begging for me, saying how sorry he was and how foolish he'd been. I took him back, and the wedding was back on. This time it stayed that way. Anyone with a brain could see this probably wasn't going to end well. People who are truly in love and want to marry one another don't usually go through that much on-again, off-again, especially when they plan to be married in only a few months. I did have a brain, but apparently I wasn't using it that day, because I married him anyway. He'd joined the military right out of high school. I graduated in June. In August, my parents and I were tired of the southern heat and we moved up north. On our drive up I stopped at the base where he was stationed, and we got married. I remember the day because I felt sick, I was scared, and I wondered just what in the world I was doing. I had an overwhelming urge to run, or lock myself in the car and not get out at the church, or do something else – anything but go in there and get married at seventeen years old to a man who had already rejected me countless times. I told myself it was just wedding jitters – the proverbial 'cold feet' – and I would be fine. I was just nervous and excited. Who wouldn't be…it was my wedding day! The only one I would ever have!

I stepped on the little voice that was my common sense talking, because I couldn't let everyone down. They expected a wedding, and they had paid for a wedding. It was short, sterile, lifeless, loveless, and to the point, and it was followed by a tiny reception in a very crowded room with my parents and Daniel's military friends. My mom was my Matron of Honor, and my dad walked me down the aisle. I don't think any of us were truly happy, deep down on the inside where it really counted. We got married in the morning, and my parents and I left that afternoon to head for the northern part of the country. Daniel had to be on base that night, anyway. We had our wedding night the night before, because that was the only night for which he could get an off-base pass. Not only did I have to ask my father's permission for that one, but when he did agree he rented us the room right next to theirs. How embarrassing and uncomfortable. The next morning, the cleaning lady walked in on us, as well. I'm not sure it could have been much more awkward, but what can you do? You have to laugh about things like that or they'll drive you crazy, make you miserable, and ruin your life – and time is way too fleeting to let that happen.

I wasn't sure when I would actually see my new husband again, but fate intervened. His father, who had been ill for some time with lung cancer, passed away, and Daniel was granted an honorable discharge from the military because he was the last male in his family who was still living. Apparently you can't be sent off to war and potentially be killed if that would wipe out your entire family bloodline on the male side. Daniel came up north, and within a week we were headed for the house in the southwest that his father had left to him. I hadn't planned to go back out west again. I couldn't imagine being away from my parents, and they couldn't imagine being away from me. Daniel had led me to believe, before the wedding took place, that we would be living wherever my parents were living. He knew I didn't want to leave them, but I think he wanted to see just how much control he had over me and how much he could get away with. I wanted to tell Daniel to forget it but I was afraid of losing him, as well. I told myself it was time to grow up and be on my own, and we left for what would now be *our* house, driving several very long days to arrive in a town I had run away from, to live in a house I had no personal interest in, with almost no money. Sound like a recipe for disaster? It was.

I talked to my parents about once a week, and I kept my calls short. There wasn't any email then, so I couldn't keep in touch that way. Daniel got angry and controlling. He thought I was spending too much time on the phone and costing him too much money. It just made me want to call more often and talk longer. He put a lock on the phone so I couldn't make long-distance calls. I had to go to a pay phone without his knowledge when he was at work to call my parents, plugging in quarter after quarter. I didn't tell them anything was wrong. I pretended I was happy, and they pretended they were happy for me.

Daniel had a good job in the medical field but he insisted I work, so I took a job at the local fast-food restaurant, and ended up working for a boy I'd had a crush on and tried to get to go out with me back in grade school. He remembered me, too. How embarrassing. And I hated the job. Being above average in intelligence can have its drawbacks. I was smarter and faster than my superiors, I learned things very quickly, and because of that everyone seemed to think I was stuck up, or that I thought too much of myself. In reality, I thought very little of myself. I only did what I did because it was easy for me to excel and I had no patience for acting in a way I perceived as stupid. I didn't know how else to be, but my own dissatisfaction with the lack of challenge at the job caused me to decide it wasn't for me. I quit, and I went to work as a waitress – with basically the same result. I had no challenge in my work, my marriage wasn't what I thought it would be, and there were always people over at our house – his friends – never a moment's peace.

After only a couple months of marriage, we started having more serious problems. I smoked at the time, and he hated it, so he started chewing tobacco and spitting in the sink and not rinsing it out – petty little things like that, but they all add up. We had been married in August, and in November I was so caught up in my misery that I allowed my mother's birthday to go by without calling her. When I realized it the next day I was mortified. I drove to a pay phone and called her up, sobbing. I felt like she would never forgive me. Of course she said it was OK, because that's what mothers do, and it was then that I told her all the things that had been going wrong and that I had been keeping to myself. I poured out my heart to her, and she wanted me to come home, but I felt I had to prove I could make my marriage work, so I stayed. It wasn't until later that my mom also confided to me how much pain my father was in. She had found him more than once, sitting on the bed in my old bedroom, his head in his hands, grieving for the loss of his daughter in his life. He wanted to follow me back out west. He didn't have to do that, because it wasn't that long before I would be headed back to the northern part of the country – but I didn't know that on the cold November day when I told my mother all my troubles.

That Christmas was the first one I ever spent away from my parents. I was eighteen years old by then, and I was miserable and resigned, and I was broke. I cashed in a couple of small savings bonds my parents had given me when I was younger in order to buy Daniel a Christmas present – an expensive gold bracelet he had been eyeing for a while. I can't remember what he bought me, and it really doesn't matter now. What matters is that the New Year came and went, and it took the last of my dignity and the chances at a good marriage with it. I moved out and stayed with a friend of mine...whom he promptly slept with. In our bed. While I was at work at some menial job. I had known her in high school and so had he, and she had always had a crush on him, but I thought nothing of it. Just like I thought nothing of one of his ex-girlfriends coming to the door to see him shortly after we arrived back in our old home town and him going outside to talk to her. Just like I thought nothing of his arrest at seventeen for allegedly abusing the girl his father had hired to cook and clean. It's amazing the things a person can ignore when she doesn't want to see what's right in front of her.

I was so desperate not to lose them that I didn't even yell about their affair. I stayed living with her...where else could I go? I gave him his wedding ring back, and said we were done, and I involved myself with one of his co-workers, Tyler. It was one of the few times in my life when I actually and actively rebelled against what I felt I 'should' do. I slept with Tyler, we went out together, we didn't even try to sneak around and be discreet. Daniel dated my 'friend' and some other people, and he wasn't much for discretion, either. We were both being manipulative and childish…just flaunting it in each other's faces. Finally, I came to my senses (through the help of my parents, of course) and decided to end the mess I was in and go back up north to be with them. I packed up and got ready to leave, but I didn't go. I made one last, futile attempt at reconciliation with Daniel. He was sitting home with a bunch of friends, playing video games on a big new TV and stereo combo he had purchased. I'm not sure where he got the money. I probably don't want to know. What I *do* know is that we allegedly never had any money when we were together, but he was the one in control of the checkbook and bank account, so how was I to know what we really had?

He didn't even pause his video game to talk to me. Obviously, our marriage meant nothing to him and my attempt at reconciliation was pointless. But I still didn't leave. I went to a friend's house and stayed there while I thought about my options. The next day, I convinced Tyler to come up north with me. He agreed. I told my parents. They said no. So I played the spoiled little bitch card; the one that had always worked for me when I was younger and didn't get my way. I told my dad that, if he didn't let Tyler come too, I wasn't coming back. What a lousy thing to do to a parent. After some discussion and a few phone calls, he agreed to construct another room on the house, where he could enclose part of the porch quite easily, to make a separate bedroom where Tyler could stay. See how dependent they were on me, too? They were willing to accept into their home – *and build a room for* – a man they had never met, simply to have their daughter back under their roof. When I look back on some of the ways I manipulated my parents in the past, it hurts my heart. But they were manipulating me, too. It was like we were all squabbling for control of everyone's life. I don't think anybody ever won. I don't even think the game was winnable.

Tyler and I drove across the country and moved in with my parents. It wasn't long before we started to fight. I wasn't happy. He wasn't happy. He couldn't seem to find a job to stick to. He missed his family. It was all very frustrating. He was a good guy overall (and he still is), but I got the feeling he was lost, and homesick, and hadn't really found his path in life just yet. The pressure of living with my parents in that tiny little room they'd made for him, and sneaking around to be with me when they were asleep, got to him. He wanted to go home to his own parents. I was so angry. Wasn't I enough for him? Apparently not, because he left. With him gone, I concentrated my efforts on making phone calls to Daniel, trying everything from begging to threatening, to get him to file for divorce so we could be well and truly done with one another. Since the last phone call I made before the divorce papers actually came in the mail I haven't spoken to him. Not once. I tracked him down through the Internet for giggles, but I have no intention of contacting him now. There's nothing there any more except a mild curiosity as to whether he would see the past the same way I do. Two people's perceptions of the same event are often radically different from one another.

In May of my eighteenth year, I received my divorce papers in the mail. I cried. I remember being so relieved it was finally over. I treated it like it was the most traumatic experience I'd ever been through, and like I had been such a victim of Daniel's cruel treatment of me. What drama! In reality, the only thing I was a victim of was my own self-deluded opinions of what my life should be like and how others should treat me. I was used to having everything basically handed to me – I'd never had to actually do anything on my own before. I think that's a lot of the reason the marriage didn't work out. Sure, we were really young, but a lot of people in generations past used to get married that young, and they made it work. They stayed together until they died. It would be easy to blame things on society and say 'Well, the world just doesn't work that way anymore. It's certainly not anything *I* did wrong.' But in reality, life is what you make of it, regardless of what society is trying to do.

We weren't committed to one another, and we weren't committed to the idea of being married. We thought it would be easy, and it wasn't. Even in the best of marriages, I don't think it's easy. Really, we had no idea what we were getting into, but I think it was especially bad because I had such a lack of understanding of what it was like to lead a 'normal' life and not be dependent on others to do everything for me. I could blame my parents for that, but I don't see the point. They obviously loved me, and they wanted to always be with me and to raise me to have as easy a childhood as possible. It's not their fault I didn't turn out quite the way they probably planned. I didn't turn out quite the way I planned, either. If it weren't for my experiences, though, I wouldn't be able to help others – which is something I didn't realize or think about when I was actually still in the experience. The philosophical thoughts about what happened to me and why only came later. I wish they would have come to me sooner, but life is a learning experience. There were certain things I had to go through to get where I needed to be. It makes sense now, but at the time I thought my life was horrible. I was needy, clingy, dependent, and depressed, and I didn't know how to change it, or even how to explain it to anyone else.

When the reality that I was finally divorced actually sunk in, I started to experience feelings of loneliness. I was back with my parents, but I wanted to fall in love and actually live happily ever after this time. I felt like a failure, and like my parents were disappointed in me. Not only had I thrown away my marriage (although I still blamed Daniel for that), but I had also thrown away my relationship with Tyler (and I blamed him for that). Instead of making sure I had a strong and healthy relationship from the beginning, I picked a relationship – any relationship I could get into – and then tried to change it to make it the 'right' relationship. I know that doesn't work. I knew it at the time, but I ignored it. We all have things we know in our hearts to be true, but sometimes we just don't want to see them or acknowledge them, so we look away and insist it will be different this time; that *we* are different; and we can make this work. It's our life, and the others around us are only supporting players. We'll have the victory because we're the star of the show. We don't stop and think about the fact that we're also the supporting players in the lives of others, whose ideas, dreams, and goals are often totally different from ours.

I went to work at a submarine sandwich shop in our small town and I actually enjoyed it, working my way up to assistant manager in short order. I started attending a local technical college and made a couple of friends there. I also dated a pot-smoking mechanic many years older than me, had a one-night stand with a college professor, and bought a motorcycle. And then I got fired from my job because I was too lazy to do enough of the work and not well-liked by the other workers, who thought I was aloof, snotty, and controlling (which I was, of course). Rebellion, all of it. Against what, I still don't know. At the time I suppose I thought it was against my parents, but I think now it might have been more against myself. I wasn't happy with who I was…didn't even really *know* who I was. Who really knows that at eighteen, anyway? I was trying to find myself. Was I the mechanic's girlfriend, enjoying the attention of a man twenty years my senior? Was I the slutty college girl, just looking for a good time? Was I the rebel on the black Kawasaki? I just didn't know.

In reality, I wasn't any of those things. Since I didn't smoke pot, that relationship ended when I asked him to choose between his drug habit and me. I cried for days over the college professor. I wanted a relationship. He wanted a one-nighter with a young girl. He won that round. I dumped the bike a couple of times because I was so afraid of it and not yet a good rider. I eventually sold it, although I often still dream of getting another one. In some less destructive ways, I'm still a secret rebel at heart. Maybe when my daughter is older and my parents are gone from this Earth I'll get another bike. Maybe not. The point, though, is that I had no identity. I was my parents' daughter, and beyond that I wasn't anyone. I tried to be Daniel's wife, and that didn't work. So I tried being Tyler's girlfriend, and that didn't work. Everything I tried seemed to blow up in my face. At the time, I wasn't able to see that I was actually the one causing this destructive pattern in my life. It was all everyone else's fault, in my opinion. That was my story, and I was sticking to it.

After several months of this I was very lonely, and I called Tyler, and we started talking. He missed me, he said, and he decided he really did want to be with me. He decided he wanted to marry me after all – something he had refused to do before, because at that time I was not a baptized Christian, and he argued that he would go to Hell if he married me. I pointed out to him that he seemed to think it was all right for him to share my bed while I was legally married to someone else, and he was a hypocrite. We had yelled at each other about that before he left the last time, and I had slapped his face and called him a bastard. Nothing seemed to faze him. Because I was desperate for his love, and because I held Christian beliefs anyway, I went and was baptized. And he still left me. Understandably, I was a bit bitter about all of that. He assured me there was *no way* he would ever do something like that again, and he was so sorry for treating me that way. I flew to Vegas, he met me there, and we were married, starting me off on marriage number two – and I wasn't even twenty years old yet.

What I Did Wrong
- Looked for someone, anyone, to marry, instead of waiting for the right person.
- Saw marriage as a validation that I was worth something and that I was 'normal,' instead of a pact between two people who love each other.
- Convinced myself that I had to fit into the mold that I thought society required for me.
- Didn't give myself enough credit for being valuable just as I was, on my own.
- Stayed in a relationship simply because I feared being alone.
- Remained in an unhealthy relationship with a friend for far too long even when it was clear she was trying to betray me.
- Let myself be brainwashed into believing things were fine in my love life when I could clearly see that they weren't.
- Shied away from the chance I had to re-invent myself and take control of my life after a cross-country move.
- Married someone I didn't even love because I didn't want to let other people down – they were expecting a wedding!

- Flaunted my affair when the marriage was in trouble, instead of keeping to myself and remaining faithful – the divorce papers hadn't even been filed yet.
- Manipulated my parents into doing things they didn't agree with just so they could have me back in their life.
- Ended up in relationship after relationship, just trying to 'be' someone and feel like I mattered to other people – that I was desirable.
- Tried to change every man I got involved with to make him into the right person for me.
- Got married a second time just because I still feared being alone and craved drama in my life.

What To Look For
- Getting married or into a serious relationship, especially at a very young age, because you don't want to be alone, not because you care about the person.
- Jumping from serious relationship to serious relationship.
- Sleeping around or dating a lot of different people at once or in rapid succession because you're desperate to find the right person.
- Picking someone because they're available and insisting you'll just change him/her to fit your needs.
- Letting others control you because you don't want to cause problems.
- Telling yourself that things are good in your relationships when all evidence clearly says otherwise.
- Being so wrapped up in your own drama that you miss out on what's around you.

What the Therapist Says
We all have an idea of how the world works. You can ask anyone about what they think is right or wrong with people or society and they will usually have an opinion. More often than not those opinions reflect whatever general views on the nature of the world the asked individual holds deep inside. Judgment is all around us. It is a most human quality, and actually necessary

for our survival. If we could not distinguish between things that are beneficial or detrimental to us we would be in a whole lot of trouble. Most of the time our ability to distinguish between the two expresses itself in whether we feel something is "good" and "right" or "bad" and "wrong." And most of the time these judgment calls do not require thought. We feel the way we feel about anything or anyone we encounter almost immediately.

But where does that automatic discrimination come from? Is there something innately "right" or "wrong" about matters, which is just obvious to all? Sadly, that does not seem to be the case. After all, things that we feel are "proper" in our society may very well be viewed negatively in another culture. If someone I am meeting for lunch continuously burps, slobbers, and makes other bodily noises while eating my immediate response will be one of disgust and aversion. But this same behavior is considered to be the epitome of respect toward the quality of the food and company in many Asian countries. The calm and quiet way we tend to associate with "fine dining" in our culture would be viewed as a terrible insult in such a country. The example illustrates that the things we grow up with, the expectations our parents, friends, and society in general express, form our concept as to how the world should work. In addition, the concept of what gives anyone "value" and "worth" is also a learned process. To some the idea that our innermost values are things we have learned can be somewhat disappointing. Personally, I see that idea as an amazing opportunity. After all, anything that has been learned can be improved upon.

How does that relate to relationship addiction? Well, the importance we put on having a relationship often stems from what we believe gives us "worth." When you think about what gives you "value," what is the first thing that comes to mind? Many immediately think of their accomplishments, their work, their successes, or the aid they give to others, their spouses and offspring. There is nothing wrong with taking pride in these. But it can become a problem if all our worth is derived from such outside sources. Sadly, much of our culture is obsessed with these external indicators of worth. We are only as good as the job we have, the clothes we wear, and whether we have a partner or family. If we think of a "family man" as opposed to a "bachelor" we value them differently in our minds. For example, if someone was to tell us his daughter was in her mid-thirties and not married many of us would immediately start wondering what might be "wrong" with her. We immediately assume some failing in those who do not fit society's expectations. In order for us to feel as if we have value we need to accomplish all those things on our internal "to do," "to have," and "to be" lists.

Another external source of worth is the feedback we get from our peers. Do you remember how scary the thought of being laughed at was, back when we were kids? We tried as hard as we could just to "fit in;" tried to change anything about ourselves in order to be accepted. Those attitudes are still with us as adults. In order to feel "right" we need to succeed in certain external ways, like having a relationship, a certain level of material wealth, and so forth. Oddly enough, even when a relationship addict achieves these things he or she will still feel "empty" inside, fearful that all that accomplishment will disappear and take the self-security away. That is the sad truth about the codependent roots of relationship addiction. It stems from an *internal* need that we unsuccessfully try to satisfy with *external* sources.

Let us assume that for some reason a young woman believes she is only worthy and acceptable as a person if she can find "someone to love her." This belief may not even be apparent to her, but sits deep in her subconscious. What kind of partner will she be drawn to? Or how about a young man who grows up believing that a "real man" has to have a lover who adores him? What might his ideal mate look like? In both cases the relationship grows from an internal need for self-validation rather than true love. The difference between the two is often hard to see, but an easy test is to ask ourselves whether we "want" to be with someone or feel that we "need" to be with someone. It sounds like such a small difference in phrasing. Yet in terms of our subconscious motivation it makes a world of difference. The concept of desperately requiring an external source of validation in order to feel "whole" is what drives codependent attitudes and lies at the root of most addictive behaviors. A person with such a mindset will eternally be on the quest for that one, perfect source of self-validation. Some turn to other addictions to numb or fill that emptiness.

Let us talk about relationship addiction in more detail. First of all, since many relationship addicts have some level of low self-esteem, this may lead the addict to believe that only a certain type of person would "want" them. So, the person in question may be willing to put up with personality traits and behaviors in his intended partner that he really does not like, but he believes this is the best he can hope for. In worse cases, such individuals may remain in openly abusive relationships simply for the deeply-held belief that this is the only person who would ever want to be with them. In cases where the addict's sense of worth is exceptionally low he or she may even see the abuse as his or her fault. The same self-blame is common to a relationship addict once the relationship ends. Even in cases where the addict is the one to end the partnership he or she will usually lay a large amount of blame on himself or herself.

It is also common for a person following the path of love addiction to immediately fill the void of a failed relationship by engaging in a new one. In some cases the seeking of a better, more "fitting" mate might even begin while the previous relationship is still going on. Finding a better partner is the means of finally feeling "whole." Rather than seeking self-worth from an inside source the focus shifts to finding "the right one," the perfect supplier for the external validation. At times this leads to a strange kind of learning process, where the addict will try out different "partner models" to discover which is the perfect fit. At other times the relationship addict might return to a previous partner since "any relationship is better than none." Whichever pattern prevails, the addict's life becomes a roller-coaster of finding and then losing new sources for emotional validation as each relationship proves as unfulfilling as the previous one.

How does one break this cycle? It may sound very abstract, but the means to do just that can be expressed in two words: Unconditional Love. It is a term often used and rarely understood. In this context I do not mean the unconditional love one person gives another but a deep-rooted love and acceptance a person has for himself or herself, no matter what the external circumstances. Our culture rarely embraces this concept, and when it does it is usually at an intellectual rather than an emotional level. How many of us honestly feel that we have unconditional value, that we are innately lovable, even if we do things wrong or are not "perfect"? I venture a guess that there are not many of us who can say we do. But, just like the subconscious beliefs that cause us pain, this can be learned. And the rewards are nothing less than miraculous.

Chapter 4: Marriage Number Two – My Daughter's Daddy

Las Vegas was great! It was August. It was 110 degrees in the shade, and Tyler was in a full tuxedo with tails. I had on a full-skirted, emerald green and black prom dress with black satin gloves that came up above my elbows. We made quite a pair, standing in line at the court house to get a marriage license, right next to the overweight couple in sweat suits and a giggling, scrawny, hippy-looking couple in tank tops, shorts, and flip-flops. The limousine driver picked us up at the hotel, carted us to the courthouse, and then drove us to the chapel. When the ceremony was over, the driver took us back to the hotel and dropped us off. I thought riding in a limo would make us look cool and classy – I thought we'd stand out, but limos are *everywhere* in Vegas. And so are wedding chapels.

If you've never been married in Vegas, allow me to enlighten you. When I got to the chapel, I was allowed to have a peek in the cooler and pick out some flowers. We showed the people at the front desk the marriage license and the rings, and they took us back to the main chapel where a preacher I had never met (no, he wasn't an Elvis impersonator) and two witnesses – women I didn't know and had never seen before – crowded around us. The ceremony lasted five minutes, and I remember giggling through most of it because the preacher was enunciating the words like a lot of the stereotypical television preachers (in the nay-ay-ay-ay-ayme of JAY-sus-ah, etc.) and Tyler and I both thought it was hilarious. As soon as it was all over and the license was signed, one woman handed me the roll of film from the camera she'd been using and the other one handed me the audio tape of the ceremony, we stopped at the front desk and paid, we changed into street clothes, and we were ushered back out the door into the stifling Vegas heat for a return limo ride to our hotel. How romantic.

That morning, getting ready for the ceremony in the hotel room we had shared the night before, I had the same sick feeling I'd experienced before my first marriage. My heart said it wasn't right. My head said it was too late now and I couldn't back out. I'd paid for the hotel and the rings, because Tyler had no money. My parents knew about the wedding – his parents did not. I'd told my parents, but hadn't 'invited' them, because I knew they wouldn't fly all the way to Vegas just for that. I remember walking in our neighborhood with my dad a few weeks earlier, asking him if he thought mom would be mad at me if I didn't have the wedding there, where we lived. Would it be OK to fly to Vegas? I only asked about mom's feelings, not about his.

Oh, I cared what he thought. I cared plenty. But I was too scared to articulate it. If I'd asked if he'd be hurt of course he'd say no, but I'd never know if he really meant it. He was pretty closed with emotions, especially when it came to his own feelings. He was raised with the belief that men didn't talk about their emotions, and they never cried. I, on the other hand, had already screwed up one marriage, and I didn't really want to talk to my dad about this next one, just in case he said something that made me feel bad or guilty.

So here I was in Vegas. I'd flown across the country. I was stuffed into a 1980s-style prom dress. There was no changing my mind – what would people think? So I told myself (again) that my fear was just wedding jitters, and it meant nothing. Tyler was so nervous he'd developed hives all over his hands and arms. He couldn't seem to stop giggling. He had lied to his parents about where he was going and why, and although I think they suspected, they couldn't prove anything and didn't question him. At the time, it never occurred to me to wonder why a twenty-five-year-old man wasn't willing to tell his parents he was getting married. I just thought it was great fun – we were getting away with something. How gleeful.

If I would've been honest with myself, I knew I was in trouble early on. When we got back to the hotel after the ceremony we decided to go get something to eat to celebrate. We had no friends or family with us, no reception, no wedding cake. We agreed we'd go and get a 'wedding pizza.' I was standing on the edge of the curb at the hotel, waiting for Tyler, who had gone to get the car he was driving – which he'd borrowed from his sister. I wasn't used to the car. I'd only seen it a couple times, and I wasn't paying attention – which I'm usually not – so I didn't really recognize him or the car when he came around the corner in it. All I saw was a sandy-haired, good looking guy in an older but well-kept sports car. I remember thinking 'Wow! That guy's *hot*!' Probably not what I should be thinking about a person who I *thought* was a stranger when I hadn't even been married an hour. Then realization set in. Oh! That's *my* hot guy. Well, that's OK then. No harm done…but I knew better than that. I just didn't want to admit it.

The plan was an exciting one: get married in Vegas, spend a little time in the desert southwest with Tyler and his family while we worked together on his motorcycle, then ride the motorcycle across the country, back to my parents' home up north. It was a great idea, with one small problem. The bike needed a lot more work than we first thought, and we had virtually no money. Oh, and I began to get my first glimpse of how…not really lazy, but just completely unmotivated, Tyler was. About anything. Because I was desperate for love and affection, and because I hadn't really spent that much actual time around Tyler for several months, and because it was amazing what I could overlook at that point in my life, I hadn't noticed this lack of motivation. I just didn't see it – or I saw it but didn't acknowledge it. Take your pick. I suppose it was a little bit of both, really.

Eventually, we gave up on the bike idea. There was no way we were going to get it ready in any kind of realistic time frame, and I was starting to suspect that Tyler might not really know what was wrong with it or how to fix it. Or maybe he just didn't have the money or the incentive. I couldn't get a straight answer, but I did get a lot of excuses. We had to get back to my parents, though, because I was beginning to feel like I was wearing out my welcome with his parents. Plus, all my things with the exception of what I could fit in a duffle bag were still at my parents' house. In order to get back cheaply, we decided to drive instead of fly. Tyler's dad let us have an older but clean and good-running vehicle that he owned as a wedding gift, we rented a small trailer for his things, and we headed out. I should have been thankful for his parents' generosity, but I felt degraded and humiliated that we weren't headed out on the bike. It was bad enough that I felt I was never good enough for my *own* parents, but now I felt inferior around *his* parents, and I was pretty sure my dad didn't really see Tyler as 'good enough' for me, even though I didn't think he would ever say so.

Eventually, we got back to the northern part of the country and my parents. We lived with them, of course. Where else would we have gone? We had no money, neither one of us had a job, and all I had was a high school education. I'd taken some college classes, but I hadn't gotten a degree. Tyler had dropped out of high school, and he didn't even have his GED. I saw no great job prospects on the horizon for either one of us. I started working at a local retail store in the mall, and my parents paid for me to go to college again, so I could try to finish my business degree. It was just a small technical college, and I was only trying for a two-year, associate's degree, but it was better than nothing, except I still didn't finish it.

It was through my job that I met Alice. She worked in the same department, and she went to the same college...I just hadn't seen her there yet. Apparently we hadn't crossed paths in the hallways. We became fast friends. She was a big girl, and very pretty in the face – like many larger women are. She looked a lot like Delta Burke from that 'Designing Women' TV show, but she had long, curly, red hair...and she was always laughing. I don't think I ever saw her angry or upset when our friendship was new, and she could make a joke out of the most troubling of circumstances. It was only once I knew her better that I saw her more serious side.

Despite our differences we were good friends. It was the first *real* friendship I think I ever had. We stuck by each other, no matter what. At school, we must have stuck by each other a bit too much, because people started to get the wrong idea. Apparently, I had a reputation I didn't even know about. Apparently, I was a lesbian. Now, I have nothing against lesbians, but I'm not one. I figured that out in high school with Margaret. I wore jeans and t-shirts. I never wore dresses. I thought a purse was an unnecessary hassle, so I just carried a man's-style wallet in my back pocket. I wore heavy, 1980's-style-black-eyeliner makeup and mismatched earrings, and my hair was short on the top and sides and long in the back. The classic 'mullet' – and a haircut favored by lesbians, I was later told. I suppose riding my motorcycle to school a couple of times didn't help, either. Never mind that the hairstyle actually looked really good on me. Never mind that I wore a wedding ring and had a husband. None of that stuff seemed to matter...or maybe people didn't even notice that part. I think they just saw the girl with the jeans and the lesbian haircut, always spending time with the dressed up, pretty, soft, giggling girl, and figured she was my girlfriend. She was. She was my girl friend. But never my *girlfriend.*

One of the things she was great about was listening to me talk (actually, complain) about my marriage. She was painfully single and wanted a husband so badly. 'Do you want mine?' I asked her. She laughed it off, until she realized I wasn't joking. We started talking more seriously about my unhappiness, and I realized something – if I wanted out, I could get out. There was no law that said I had to remain married. The main problem was what my parents would think. Would they think I was stupid? Would they feel as though they'd failed me? Would they turn their backs on me? How could I make it out to be Tyler's fault (which of course it really was anyway, I told myself), so that mommy and daddy would still love me, and not blame me? I had to think about that, but one thing was clear: I was unhappy, and manipulative enough to change things in my favor.

To top it all off, my parents wanted to move back to the South. They said the northern winters were too cold. It was too much for them as they got older, and they couldn't take all the cloudy days. It was turning my father into an old man. His hands were starting to tremble and he was beginning to look his age, for the first time in his life. It scared me. Despite the conflicting emotions I sometimes had about my parents, there was no question about loving them. That was never an uncertain thought. That was my daddy, and I couldn't imagine him not being there. My mom didn't take the cloudy days as hard, but she was still unhappy. She was tired a lot, and not in the best of moods. It was clear that neither one of them was pleased with where we were living.

Alice and I hatched a plan. I would get a divorce, my parents could move, and she and I would get an apartment together. I was really scared at the thought of living away from my parents, but I was exhilarated, too. Finally, I could prove that I could survive on my own! I could have a life that was really *mine*, instead of one that was carefully constructed to be what I thought others wanted me to have – what was expected of me. I told Tyler I wanted out, I told my parents of the plan to live with Alice, and they were shocked that I would end another marriage and skeptical that Alice and I could afford to live on our own. I showed them apartment prices and job listings in the paper, and told them how we could do it. They decided they would postpone their move for a few months, to see if Alice and I really could get those jobs and an apartment, and if we could keep them and pay our bills. I just knew we could do it. But before we got a chance, something else happened.

At that point in my life I had basically no money, a dead-end job, and I was bored with my college classes. They were taking too long and they were too easy, and I was getting really tired in them, almost falling asleep at my desk. I didn't know why I was so tired all of a sudden, but I put it down to stress over my unhappy marriage and trying to pretend like everything was OK. I was wrong. About six months into our marriage, and about a month after the tiredness started, I fell asleep sitting up in one of my classes and my head jerked forward so hard it almost bounced off the desk. That was bad, and I was starting to get scared. What if there was something really wrong with me? I'd always been anxious, and my thoughts tried to run away with me. What if it was cancer, or a heart problem, or…? I just didn't know, but I tried not to say anything about it to anyone else. I didn't want to worry them. I thought it would go away, but it didn't, and I started to get nauseated very easily. In the meantime, Tyler and I decided we were definitely going to split up, and I told my parents we were planning to get a divorce. Neither one of us wanted to be married to the other one anymore. It wasn't anything like we thought it would be.

Later that week, when Tyler hadn't left to move back in with his parents yet and we were still making arrangements to file for divorce, I was looking at the calendar and I suddenly had a scary thought…I was two weeks late. What if I was pregnant? Was *that* why I was so tired? That couldn't be…could it? We were usually pretty careful, and since we didn't get along that well there hadn't been that much to be careful *of*. I didn't say anything to Tyler. I didn't want to scare him for nothing, and it was probably nothing. Plus, if it wasn't nothing, I wasn't sure what I was going to do, or what he would think. It was easier to keep quiet. I told my mother my theory but she shrugged it off. No way. I jokingly bet her five dollars that I was, and she went and bought me a test. I remember sitting alone in the bathroom on the closed toilet lid, waiting for the test to be finished. Mom was the only one who knew. I still hadn't said anything to Tyler, and I certainly hadn't said anything to my father. As far as he knew, I was planning a second divorce. I stood up to look at the test when the time was up. When I saw the two blue lines I sat back down, hard, and put my head between my knees, trying not to pass out while my ears rang and the world spun all around me. I was pregnant. Mom never did give me the five dollars, but considering I had no money and no insurance and my parents paid for everything, I shouldn't complain.

In my mind at that time, it was the worst thing that could have *ever* happened to me. I wanted a divorce, not a baby! I wanted my freedom back, to go and be someone else. Now, even if I got divorced, I'd never be free. Unless I had an abortion. No matter what, I had to go to the doctor. And I had to tell Tyler. I didn't want to. I wanted to simply divorce him and never tell him anything. Unless... What if I did have the baby? What if we stayed together? I could have what society said was a *real* life. A husband, a child. Maybe he and I could eventually get along better, and get our own place, and maybe we could be happy after all. My thoughts on the matter changed so very quickly. I went from *hating* the idea to thinking it was a great opportunity in the space of about twenty minutes. I went into our bedroom, and I lay down on the bed, and I stared at the ceiling. Tyler wandered in and sat down and just looked at me for a while.

"You're pregnant, aren't you?" he finally asked.

I nodded, and he sighed and didn't say anything. Once Tyler knew I sat up on the bed and looked at him.

"Can we keep it?" I asked, already thinking about everything we could plan for: the cute and tiny clothes and all the rest.

He looked back at me calmly. "It's not a puppy."

I was shocked. This was our *child*. How could he say that? I cried, and I cajoled, and I made promises I knew I would never keep. To this day, I really couldn't even tell you why I did it. I hadn't wanted the baby, but once he said he didn't, keeping it was all I could think about. Some of it was probably pregnancy hormones, but most of it was just me – I was so confused that I didn't even realize it. I thought everything I was thinking was completely rational. In truth, I was so far off rational I was coming back around to it from the other direction. It's hard, even now, to explain why I did things the way I did them.

I was torn between wanting my freedom and wanting the kind of life that society always told me I was supposed to have. It was programmed into me that having 2.5 kids, a dog, and a station wagon was the American way. It was just what people *did.* What kind of person would I be if I turned my back on that? I didn't know which idea was right for me, or would finally make me happy, and I was terrified beyond belief to choose, so I was wildly oscillating between the two. I convinced Tyler to keep the baby. I convinced him we would stay together and make it all work out. He even called his parents and told them about it. They were ecstatic. My parents had much the same reaction. They were going to be grandparents, and since I was their only child, this was a huge moment for them. I'll never forget how happy they looked when they heard the news.

Even with the coming baby, Tyler and I continued to fight, and everything continued to deteriorate. We couldn't agree on anything to do with our relationship and future, and we couldn't agree on anything to do with the baby. That was it. This was ridiculous. Enough was enough. I *really* wanted out, and I tried to wait and see if it got better, but it didn't. A couple of weeks was hardly enough time to change things, but I had no patience with anything. I wanted what I wanted, and I wanted it *now*. A few days later I broke my parents' hearts by coming to them and telling them I wanted an abortion, and I wanted to go ahead with the divorce. My father, a pained look in his eyes, told me he would never understand, but he would pay for it if that was what I really wanted. He knew I had no money to pay for the procedure. He had a hand on my shoulder as we stood there talking, and I was close enough to see how defeated he looked. I knew how much he loved me, but I could see the disappointment mixed in there, as well. This was his chance to have a grandchild, and he'd been thinking about it for days, and now I had come along and said that it wasn't happening after all, because I was too selfish. I felt like a terrible person. I didn't understand how anyone could love me, or how I could be worth anything to anyone. I guess I didn't see the point in much of anything, really.

My marriage – and my second one, at that – was no good. My parents had to hate me by now – I was just a big disappointment to them. I was carrying around a tiny, accidental life that I didn't even want and was too wrapped up in my own problems to keep. Everything in my life was wrong and going more wrong by the minute. I went to the doctor, and during the examination he said that something didn't feel right. Great. More good news. He was afraid I might have an ectopic pregnancy, where the baby has implanted outside of the uterus, in a fallopian tube. It's sometimes called a tubal pregnancy, and if I did have one I'd have to go to surgery, right then, or I could die. I'd been afraid of death since my earliest memories, and that fear hadn't lessened with age. I was sent across to another complex at the hospital, where I had to drink an enormous amount of water and then be screened through ultrasound technology in order to see what was what. In addition to being miserable I was terrified, and my bladder was rapidly nearing capacity. My mother waited out in the hall while I was thoroughly examined.

I came out half an hour later, sobbing. She feared the worst. She knew how deeply frightened I was of anything medical, especially surgery. I sat down next to her, and I poured out my heart, telling her over and over again how I *had* to keep it. The technician had shown me a perfect little jelly bean shape, miniscule hands folded in by its chest and a strong heartbeat. It had only been around for 6.3 weeks, but it was already a living creature in its own right, and it was beautiful and perfect. It deserved a chance. I know there are people out there who would disagree, and say that life begins at birth, not conception. You keep your opinions, and I'll keep mine, and we'll agree to disagree. To me, what I saw was a brand new *life*. How could I just kill it because I was selfish and spoiled? So what if it wasn't planned? An accident and a surprise are not the same thing.

From that moment on, the word 'abortion' was never mentioned again, unless it was preceded by the words "I'm so glad I didn't get an…" In my head and in my heart, I rededicated myself to my marriage, such as it was, and I was even happy for a while, fascinated by what I had seen on that ultrasound screen. It's an image I'll take to my grave. Then I started throwing up every morning, which didn't make me happy at all, but eventually I got used to it and about the time I adjusted to my new morning routine, the nausea just faded away. We continued to live with my parents, and we continued to work at our menial jobs, and we continued to argue, only not as much as we used to. Originally, neither one of us had wanted a child, but we were slowly warming to the idea that this might be something really worthwhile. It could very well be the most important thing we would ever do with our lives, and we didn't want to screw it up.

Since there would be no apartment for Alice and I, and since my parents still wanted to relocate to a warmer climate, and since Tyler and I were at least going to be together for a while, I said my goodbyes to Alice and my old life in the North and Tyler and I moved with my parents. The Deep South, where I had experienced my senior year of high school, was my parents' choice, and we rented a mobile home there until we found a place that my parents wanted to buy. I drove my mother's car all the way from near the Canadian border, big pregnant belly and all. I was six months along by then, and I was starting to waddle. I wasn't sure the heat of a southern summer would be the best choice, but what could I do? The die was cast. I was excited, and it was a new adventure. I wasn't much for sitting around with no drama in my life. There always had to be something. Routine was just not me…but when I was feeling anxious or nervous routine was what I fell into, so I was back and forth like a yo-yo, probably even more than I realized. Others had trouble figuring me out because of it, and I had trouble figuring me out, as well.

Even though I was 'happy' with my choice, my thoughts still often strayed to other pursuits, other ideas, other lives. What would I do, really, if I could do anything? I just didn't know. I wasn't sure whether I could ever really be away from mom and dad, or whether I even wanted to be. They always did so much for me that I didn't know how *not* to rely on them. I didn't know how to be self-sufficient, and I went back and forth from wanting to run far away to wanting to never leave, over and over and over again. It's a background pattern that has pervaded my entire life from my earliest memories until the writing of these words, over thirty years later. It is always there.

Finally, with the baby almost ready to arrive, Tyler and I got our own place...sort of. My parents had purchased a five-acre tract of land, on which sat a rather decrepit and small mobile home. It wasn't falling down or dangerous, but it was clearly old and needed some upgrading – or a bulldozer. We all lived in it for a few weeks until they bought a larger and newer mobile home, and they had it moved onto the same five acres. They moved to that one, and they gave us the old one. We did what we could to make it a home. It consisted of three tiny bedrooms and two cramped baths, but it really had everything we needed. It also had a lot of roaches, and the floor would run away from us when we turned on the kitchen light at night. I couldn't bring a baby into that! Some well-placed bait had me sweeping up literally dustpans full of roaches in the morning for probably a week or more. After that we really had no more problems with insects, and we made up a little nursery in the smallest bedroom with second hand furniture bought at yard sales, and thrift store blankets and baby clothes. It wasn't the life I had envisioned for myself, but it wasn't all bad. At least we had a place to live and I was having an easy pregnancy. Still, I couldn't escape the thought that I was only playing house, not really 'living' – I wasn't being true to myself.

I had some much-wanted freedom back, because Tyler took a job with a trucking company. He was gone most of the week, and then he slept almost all weekend while he was home. This was terrible when I was lonely, but great when I wanted to do my own thing...although I was becoming increasingly awkward and tired as my belly expanded. I stayed home more and more. We didn't have much money, and neither one of us had much energy. In mid-October of that year he was on a run up in Northern Alabama, and I was playing cards with my parents after dinner. We were all laughing and listening to the radio and having a great time. Eventually, I became aware that my stomach hurt. Must have been something I ate, because it was fading away now...and now it was back. Uh-oh. Labor pains? But it was ten days early! I wasn't ready! I just kept playing cards, and

I didn't say anything. Surreptitiously, I looked at my watch. The pains were about nine minutes apart, so there was no need in alarming anybody just yet. They might stop on their own. I went home at about eight that night, walking the 100 feet or so across the yard to my own little place and packing my hospital bag. Then I tried to sleep.

Sleep was elusive, and I had a million thoughts going through my head. What if something went wrong? What if I slept soundly and woke up and it was time and I had to have the baby right there in my bed? What if, what if, what if…? The 'what ifs' were a big part of my life. I had them when I was a kid, and I have them now. They never completely go away, but they were extra-strong that night as I lay in bed, all alone, desperately wanting company but not wanting to disturb anyone. I didn't want to be a bother. Hadn't my tumultuous life caused my parents enough trouble already? Finally, at about six the next morning, I made my way over to my parents' home and let myself in. I sat quietly on the love seat while they still slept. Just knowing that someone was close by was helpful, but I was still scared.

When I had first decided to keep the baby it was exciting, but it was the *idea* of the baby – and that ultrasound picture – that had kept me going. The idea of actually *having* the baby – of going through labor and delivery – was easy to think about because it was a long way away. I'm ashamed to admit this but in the spirit of honesty, I will: Part of the reason I originally stuck with my decision to keep the baby after the initial joy of the ultrasound pictures wore off was because I wouldn't have to worry about it for several months. If I had the abortion I had to do it right then, and I was afraid of it. Now that I was having labor pains and the reality of what was going to happen was starting to set in, I was frightened beyond belief at the unknown of what I would have to go through. It didn't help that my doctor was young, male, and incredibly good looking. How embarrassing.

My mother got up at about six-thirty, and when she came out of the bedroom into the living room, she froze in her tracks at the sight of me on her love seat.

"Is it time?" she whispered, and when I nodded she stuck her head back into the bedroom and awakened my dad. Everybody tried to stay calm, but of course you can't really do that too well when there's a baby on the way, now can you? Mom took me to the doctor's office when it opened at eight and he said that yes, I was in early labor, and no, it wasn't a big deal, and I should come back either (a) when my water broke, or (b) when the contractions were four minutes apart, whichever happened first. With mom driving, I went to Tyler's work and picked up his paycheck and asked his boss if he could get a message to him. I went to the bank. I went back to the doctor with four-minute-apart contractions and they said I could just go to the hospital whenever I was ready, or I could wait until my water broke. I went to my father's furniture store and hung out for a while. I went to dinner with my family, even though I could only drink a soda – I wasn't allowed to eat while I was in labor. Finally, at about seven that night, I got bored and checked into the hospital and they broke my water for me and we were underway. I missed Tyler. Despite the fact that we often fought and really didn't get along well even when we weren't fighting he was about to be a father, and I didn't want him to miss that.

As it turned out, I didn't need to worry. His boss had gotten a message to him, and he made it there just minutes before the actual delivery got started. He was exhausted and dirty and smelled like diesel fuel but he was there, and at that moment I needed him. My mom and dad were also there. Dad wasn't going to come in, but the nurse saw that he was wearing a path in the hallway, so she told him he'd better just come in the room. Back in his day men didn't do that, so it was all new to him, but he got to see his first and only grandchild come into this world, and once she was cleaned up and checked out and pronounced healthy, he got to carry her down to the nursery for the first time. He still insists she was 'no bigger than a peanut,' but having actually expelled her from my body, I beg to differ. My beautiful little girl, Karyn Elizabeth, came into the world just after one-thirty in the morning, and I stayed the rest of the night at the hospital, Tyler sleeping on a cot in my room. Both my daughter and I went home the next day.

For a little while, life was pretty good. I felt like I was doing what I was 'supposed' to be doing – staying married, having a baby, making a 'normal' life for myself. It was all an act. I was playing a part, and in my mind I was often somewhere else – some*one* else. But I was glad I had my daughter. Now that it was done and I could look upon her delicate and perfect little face as she slept, I had no regrets about having a child – but I still wasn't happy overall. The 'standard' that society seemed to want me to meet just wasn't me. I wasn't really wife and mother material. I didn't know how to change a diaper or heat up a bottle or make baby formula. Tyler had to teach me all that, and my mom helped me learn how to hold my daughter right so I wouldn't hurt her. I got little sleep. Tyler went back to his truck driving job just a few days after she was born, and I took care of the tiny infant.

I ended up spending most nights sleeping at my parents' house, terrified that little Karyn might stop breathing during the night, and when I woke up and found her dead in her crib, there would be no one there to help me. No one to hear my anguished screams. It was a sick and morbid thought, but I couldn't get it out of my head. It was another one of those 'what ifs' that just wouldn't leave me alone. I would sneak over to her crib during the night and wiggle her just a bit so she'd move, and I could feel safe again. Sometimes I startled her and she started crying, and then I had to stay up…and I was angry with her for making noise and keeping me awake. People who have never had children don't realize how incredibly sleep-deprived you actually get, and how short your temper can be. Add to that how spoiled I was and how used to mommy and daddy always taking care of everything, and it was a real shock to have to care for this tiny, wriggling, screaming creature that didn't give a damn *how* tired I was.

Less than three weeks after she was born, I turned twenty-one years old. Tyler was on the road. I really didn't have any friends, so there was no real party. Just me and mom and dad and my daughter, a small cake, and whatever I wanted to eat for dinner that night. Not exactly what I expected my life to be like. When I was little, I had wanted to be a marine biologist, swimming around under the sea studying strange and wonderful creatures. Just before I found out I was pregnant I was taking flying lessons, doing stalls at several thousand feet in the air, climbing a ladder to fuel the plane, de-icing before takeoff and spending time in ground school, learning about the mechanics of flight – I wanted to be a pilot. For a while I had wanted to be a motorcycle mechanic, and then a truck driver, or a diesel truck mechanic, a construction worker, or maybe a race car driver. All unconventional jobs for a woman, certainly, but I was (and still am) an unconventional woman. I knew I was different, and I was trying to fit in with society, and it was like two great, opposing forces grinding against one another. I didn't know which would break first – society's hold on who and what I 'should' be, or my spirit…and it was terrifying. I never felt so amazingly happy and yet so completely and utterly trapped as I did when I looked upon my sleeping daughter's face, or reflected on how she relied on me for everything. Assuming no one jumped in to help if I neglected her, she would simply die. Without me, she would cease to be. The responsibility of that was overwhelming.

It wasn't long before she started to grow and develop, and she was able to crawl and then to walk on her own. She got into everything, she smiled and giggled at me, and she seemed to be really *aware* of what was going on around her. Children of that age are still young enough to be amazed by their world, and not yet aware of all of the ugliness that lies within it. They see only the beauty, and they are both fascinat*ed* by their world, and fascinat*ing* to observe. I'd like to say I really spent the time that I should have with my daughter, and I'd like to tell you a story of happily-ever-after, but I can't – not and keep any shred of honesty. Tyler and I continued to fight, and I continued to do everything I could to make it look like it was always his fault, no matter who started it.

He spent very little time with our daughter, even when he was home. As a result, I felt put-upon and like I was expected to do everything. In reality, I didn't have it that bad. My mother made dinner for all of us every night, and she helped make formula and sterilize bottles and wash clothes and change diapers. She was there for me and for my daughter, and so were my dad and my uncle Bernie, my mom's brother. He was one of the good guys. I grew up spoiled, and I still wasn't used to not having everything handed to me, so I of course complained. The only real reason I had to complain was that Tyler wasn't there much, either for me or for our child. He slept a lot, and he didn't seem to take much interest in anything. He even quit truck driving and took a job closer to home at my insistence, but things didn't improve.

It wasn't long before he was becoming fast 'friends' with the girls he worked with at an elder care facility and I was talking to a guy who he used to work with at a hardware store. Both were innocent from a physical standpoint, but not so much from an emotional one. There was too much speculation involved. This was mostly on my part (I was bored with him already), but there was some on his part, as well. Later on, he admitted kissing one of the women at his work, who allegedly forced herself on him. Since Tyler was well over six feet tall I found it hard to believe that he couldn't have said no, but that doesn't matter much anymore. I wasn't even that upset about it. While he was going through his own thing, I was doing essentially the same thing, only worse. At my father's suggestion I decided to get into real estate. I saw dollar signs – the housing market was growing. I took a class to get certified…and slept with my instructor. Yes, I knew he was married. I thought he would leave his wife, like so many 'other women' do, and I had the drama back in my life again. Look what I was getting away with!

Do you want to know the worst thing? I didn't even like him that much…and I certainly wasn't in love with him. He was overweight and not very cute and clearly just looking for someone other than his wife to have sex with. All that mattered to me was that he paid attention to me. After a few rendezvous after class, I wanted more of a real relationship and he wouldn't give it and that was the end of that. I used to drive by his house, just to see if he was home, even after it was all over. I kept thinking he'd call me and tell me that he realized he loved me and he was leaving his wife…and this was a man *I didn't even want!* Eventually I got over it and got an actual real estate job with a different agency, and I got involved with a (married) agent who was almost forty years older than me, and then with the owner of the agency. He was also married, and he wasn't happy with his situation. While we never actually had sex, we were certainly well past the point of being friends and colleagues.

Working in real estate was a great way to cheat on a spouse…not that I'm recommending that!…because it was so easy for me to call Tyler and say I was showing a house. He didn't know where I was, and that kind of power over another person and the deception that came along with it was something I really enjoyed. It was just another version of the 'act' that I put on as a wife and mother. It was like playing a role – it wasn't really me, but I could pretend it was for a while because it worked for what I wanted to accomplish at the time. One night Tyler was in town for some reason and he drove by the real estate office and my car was there, so he stopped in. While he didn't actually catch us doing anything I'm sure we looked guilty, and he definitely suspected something.

I had to get away from the agency and real estate in general – not because I felt bad for doing something wrong, but because I feared getting caught. I didn't want to be made to be 'the bad guy.' I couldn't allow that. I was already planning ways to adjust the situation so Tyler and I wouldn't be together much longer, and there was no way I could let that look like my fault, either to anyone else or to myself. There are things you really *know,* deep down inside, and there are things you tell yourself to get by. I lived in that 'tell yourself to get by' world for a long time, and I almost managed to convince myself that it was real. Eventually, the deep-down knowing would creep into my thoughts, and I couldn't always push it away. It was during those times I felt most alone and most worthless, but I tried to hide it behind anger at other people, and what *they* were (supposedly) doing to harm me.

Tyler and I separated – not a big surprise, really, but made more complicated because we had a child. Our daughter Karyn and I lived in the little, run-down trailer that we had called home. Because he had nowhere to go, Tyler lived in a bedroom at my parent's house. Why didn't I move in with my parents? No way! I wasn't giving up the freedom that I thought I was getting back, and I certainly wasn't giving Tyler the trailer. Around this same time my friend Alice from up north got in touch with me, and she had to have some pretty serious surgery. She said she knew I couldn't afford to be there, but she wanted to let me know. I left at seven at night, and I drove straight through – over fourteen hours – to be there the morning of the day before surgery. Deeply touched, she spent the day with me and I was there the next day when she went to the hospital and was one of the first people to see her when she woke up. She did just fine. While I was there I met one of her friends, Maximillian, whom I instantly liked.

He was short, and cute, and nicely built. Green-eyed and with almost white-blonde hair, he looked like a California surfer, not a northern-US native. He and I went to dinner while Alice was in the hospital. He refused to get involved with a married woman, which made me want him that much more. We always seem to want what we can't have, don't we? I had to go back to the South, and we said our goodbyes. We wrote letters and called each other quite often, and he seemed to really like me. He agreed to come and see me if and when I was actually single. Even knowing I was separated from my husband was not enough for him, and while I respected it, it also drove me crazy. I *had* to have him, and that meant I *had* to get free of Tyler.

We filed for that inevitable divorce, and Tyler was given visitation rights and ordered to pay child support. I had physical custody of Karyn. Nobody paid anybody any alimony, and none of us had legal fees, because we hadn't bothered to get lawyers. We just bought the papers and filled them out and carried them down to the courthouse and filed them, and then got an appointment to go before the judge. Getting divorced in this country is pathetically easy, and I'm not so sure that's a good thing. Naturally, when you want a divorce it's great, but…well, society's just changing a lot. I only found out later how much Tyler cried, and for how long, after it was over. I didn't know at the time about the drinking or the depression. No one else told me, and Tyler certainly wasn't going to. I wasn't aware of the fact I had broken his heart, and I can't say for sure whether I would have really cared if I *had* known at the time. Cruel, but true. I care *now,* of course, but then again, I'm really not the same person I was then.

Not long after the divorce I got a new mobile home. Brand new. It wasn't very big, and it wasn't very fancy, but it was new and it was mine. Some people came and hauled the old one away and put the new one in place and hooked everything up for me. I had actually wanted to move half an hour or so away and rent an apartment, but my parents talked me out of it. My dad didn't seem to think I could do it, but maybe he was just concerned for me. I had gotten a job in a neighboring city, and my boss wouldn't even let me have the day off to see them put my new house in. I almost quit over that because I thought my boss was a royal bitch anyway, but I knew I could lose the trailer if I didn't have a job and couldn't pay the bills. What would my parents think if I did that? I'd be a disappointment to them yet again. I already had two divorces behind me. I already had a baby, and I was only twenty-three years old. I already felt like a huge failure. I already felt like I couldn't do anything right. I already felt worthless. I had my freedom back in the sense that I wasn't married anymore, but who was going to want me now that I had a child? Not a lot of men wanted a 'package deal,' and this was especially true of men in their early to mid-twenties. So. I was stuck again. Trapped…just in a different way this time.

I felt like maybe my life was getting back on track when I found out more about the ex-friend of Tyler's, Lee, who worked at the hardware store and who I'd been talking to, on and off when I saw him around, for a while. He had kids! Two kids, a boy and a girl, with two different ex-wives…*and* he had custody of both of them. I thought he must be a great father. I never stopped to think that maybe the mothers were horrendous people and he was simply the lesser of two evils, or that maybe the mothers didn't even want their kids. The first time he asked me out, he was drunk. I said no. Finally I accepted his phone number, and after a few days I called him. He was drunk. There seemed to be a pattern there but I didn't want to see it, so I ignored it. Instead of saying he was an alcoholic and I'd be wise to stay away from him, I said he was a poor, misguided, pained soul who needed someone to care about him. I really still liked Maximillian, but he was 1000 miles away from me and I was lonely. I started dating Lee because he was there, and because he was fun. He drank a lot but he was a happy drunk, so he was always enjoyable to be around.

While my mom and dad watched my daughter I went out more and more often to bars with Lee where we drank and smoked and shot pool and danced and listened to the juke box late into the night. Since I worked retail I didn't have a 9-to-5 schedule, and I had the chance to pretty much do what I wanted. I didn't see myself as out of control, or neglectful of my child, or any of that. I see it now, but then...all I saw then was that I was having a good time and it couldn't really be wrong if *I* was doing it. I was conceited, and arrogant, and haughty on the outside, and on the inside I was a withering little child, frightened of my own shadow and desperate for love and attention – but only on my terms. I worked hard to hide it and act like life was wonderful, but it wasn't easy. I started to get depressed, lethargic, and easily upset. I also started getting desperate for more of Lee's attention. It didn't seem like I was able to 'fix' him, but I wanted to. I cared – really *cared* – very much for him, and it hurt me that I couldn't make everything better.

We were on-again, off-again for several months, and there was always drama. I said I hated it, and I complained about it daily, but deep down I craved it. It was exciting and different, and there was always something new going on. While all that was going on, Maximillian was still calling me and sending me letters. I had gotten divorced, which was what he said he was waiting on, but he couldn't just run to the South. He didn't have much money and he was in college and had a job as well. Eventually, he saved up enough money to come to see me, but by then I was already wrapped up in my dealings with Lee. Maximillian came down anyway because the trip was already booked, but I refused to see him because I was dating Lee. It was a crappy thing to do. It was mean, and it was cruel. I'm sure he thought so, too. I don't really know whether he had a good time in my state or not, but he seemed to be his usual happy self overall the next time I talked to him on the phone, even though there was a bit of an edge to his voice that I hadn't noticed before.

He was hard to read sometimes. He acted like nothing bothered him, but I'm sure it really did. You'd think I would've been flattered by all the attention, too, but I just found it annoying. I was trying to be a one-man woman with Lee and here Maximillian was, nagging me about getting together for lunch. Couldn't he see I was busy? I had moved on from him. Even after he went home to the North he still kept calling me and talking to me. I finally sent him a letter saying that I didn't want to see him. Period. He got the letter on Christmas Eve, after he had already mailed me a beautiful necklace, and sent a ring for my daughter as well. Real gold, not cheap stuff. It hadn't come in until after I mailed the letter out. I didn't return either piece of jewelry, even after Alice called me and told me how hurt Maximillian was and that it was a terrible thing I did. She and I didn't speak much for a while after that, but I soon shoved it to the back of my mind. I was busy with Lee.

One night shortly after all that happened with Maximillian's wasted trip, I met up with Lee at our favorite little local bar. It was actually a great hangout. No one really expected you to drink a lot, there was no pressure to be someone you weren't, and it was never very crowded. It was just a little corner country bar where all the locals knew each other, and there was always a pool table open. I pulled into the parking lot, and Lee came walking out to meet me. He had already gotten a good start on the evening's alcohol intake. Where I drank no more than three beers when we went out, and usually only had one or two, he drank ten or twelve in that same time period – and he was a couple of inches shorter than me, weighing about the same as I did. He wrapped his arms around me, beer bottle still in one hand, and put his head on my shoulder, clinging to me like I was his last hope. He was close to crying. When I asked him what was wrong, he just shook his head. I asked him again, and he pulled away just enough to be able to look into my eyes and told me that he was never going to love me. It just wasn't there, and he was so, so sorry.

I didn't know what to do. I mean, what do you say to something like that? I knew I didn't want to lose him...maybe I could change his mind some day. After all, how do you *know* that you'll never love someone? Maybe you just don't love them *yet.* Of course he would love me...I just had to be patient and give it some time. I told myself that, and I told him that...sort of.

107

I didn't think a big speech would work, so I just told him he didn't have to love me. He could just like me and we could date and have fun together and there was no pressure. Inside I was crushed, but on the outside I kept pretending like everything was fine. So we stayed dating...for a little while. I eventually stopped seeing him under pressure from my parents (big surprise there, right?) because they didn't like him and thought he drank too much.

Around that time one of my acquaintances had also introduced me to Mike, who was a police officer, and my parents liked him right away. Clean-cut, respectable job, no alcohol, etc. I started seeing him instead of Lee, but my heart just wasn't in it. He just wasn't as much fun. He only wanted to talk about how great he was and how nice his car was and things like that, and he was incredibly condescending on top of it. It soon got old.

He thought my brand new trailer was terrible. After all, hadn't I ever heard the term 'trailer trash'? It wasn't good enough. Didn't I want something better? He didn't seem to understand I was happy. It wasn't about material things. They just weren't that important to me. I thought I could be a good person without fortune or fame, but Mike disagreed. I don't even really think it was about me. I think it was about him, and how he didn't want to be associated with a girl who wasn't rich and perfect. The truth was, he wasn't rich either – he lived with his mother! All that luxury and that big, beautiful house didn't even belong to him, and he had the nerve to look down on *me,* and what I *owned,* and what I was *working for*, just because I didn't live a high-dollar lifestyle.

I don't think your bank account really has much to do with the quality of your life, as long as you have a roof over your head and enough to eat. I think the way you look at things has a lot more to do with whether you feel your life is worthwhile. Of course, at that time I didn't feel that way – I just felt bad. Once again, I was judged to be 'not good enough' by someone I liked – or at least my parents liked him, so I figured I was supposed to like him as well – it would make them happy. Even when he stood them up the night they bought dinner for all of us and brought it to the house, they still liked him. They just shrugged it off and said it was no big deal. I was outraged. He didn't feel like coming by, and he didn't feel like calling, either, so he just didn't. Nice guy. He thought he was better than us, and he didn't even have the decency to try to hide that.

He went back and forth between being possessive and controlling, and being completely unavailable. After a while, I felt like he was playing a game with me, and I started to be afraid of him. He carried a gun for work, and often showed up at my house in uniform unannounced...I think he did it mostly because he was on a power trip. At first I found it sexy, then routine, then frightening. I was grateful we only dated for a short time. Who knows what he might have done if I'd let him gain any more control over my life. I was headed into that pattern of the woman who just takes the abuse because she doesn't think she's worth anything more than that, but I hadn't gotten so far down that path that I was lost. Instead I got pissed off, and I rebelled.

One night, a few short weeks after he stood my parents up for dinner, Mike went to the house of some friends of ours, which happened to be right down the street from Lee's house. I had given in...called up Lee and told him how much I missed him, and we had gotten back together. My car was out front, and it was pretty late at night. Mike saw my car at Lee's house and had a fit. My parents had a fit. My friends had a fit. They all had the same fit – one of the "what the *hell* were you thinking?" variety. All I was thinking was that I just wanted to be happy, and I had much more of that with Lee than with Mike. He might drink too much, but he was always fun and always kind and never treated me badly or made me feel like I wasn't good enough. He was, despite his drinking, a truly good person in many ways. I don't know where he is now. Sometimes I wish I did, but you can't go home again.

The eventual pressure of my parent's displeasure and Lee's drinking led us to part company for good. My parents didn't shun me, but their comments about Lee's problem increased, as did the thinly-veiled remarks about my lack of attention to my daughter. Was I going out *again* tonight? I tried to push it to the back of my mind but it wasn't easy, and I found a reason to pick a fight with Lee, so I could break it off. I didn't want to do that, but I felt like I had to choose between my parents and Lee, and I had too much loyalty to my parents to turn my back on them for a man. I was weak, and I wasn't brave enough to stand up for myself where my parents were concerned, for fear they might not be there for me any more if I spoke my mind. I guess in a way I was brainwashed, but whether they did it or whether I simply did it to myself I don't really know.

I missed Lee, and I was miserable. I wasn't about to try to get back in touch with Maximillian and grovel for his attention, and I couldn't imagine anyone else ever wanting me now that I was twice-divorced with a young daughter. To try to cheer me up, a friend took me to a Country-Western bar in a neighboring town, where I met another man. I hadn't intended to find someone else. I wasn't even looking. That didn't matter, though, because once I saw him, he was all I could see. I wasn't good at being without a relationship, and I always felt like I didn't even matter unless I mattered to someone else. I knew I mattered to my parents, but as I got older that didn't seem to be enough for me. I was all grown up now. A woman. And what kind of woman was I without a man? Now, here I was in a country bar with my eye on a redneck guy. My parents were country people, so how could they possibly object to a country boy? Time for another pursuit. What I didn't know at the time, though, was how deep I was getting myself in, and how much of a toll this new relationship would take my both my mental and physical health – and the health and happiness of my tiny daughter.

What I Did Wrong
- Married someone just to get married again – for the drama, or to try to prove a point.
- Made a weak attempt at breaking free of parental control by getting married in Vegas.
- Missed the 'red flag' of Tyler not telling his parents about the wedding – they didn't even know we were engaged!
- Gave up (again) and let my parents control what I did instead of standing up for myself.
- Rebelled and acted underhandedly and sneakily instead of being honest about my unhappiness.

- Let my spoiled attitude get in the way of the care I should have been giving my daughter.
- Chose to keep a baby instead of having an abortion because 'I wouldn't have to deal with it for a while.' While I'm grateful every day to have my daughter, I originally decided to keep her for entirely the wrong, selfish reason.
- Treated someone horribly after he made an effort to come see me and reach out to me, because 'I couldn't be bothered.'
- Gave up and got divorced instead of working on my marriage, just because things weren't perfect.
- Had my eye on other men while I already had one, and couldn't settle on any of them – probably because the feelings that should have been there weren't there for any of them.

What To Look For
- Wanting what you don't have and hating it (or getting bored with it) as soon as you've gotten it.
- Dating/marrying just to make someone else happy (or just to anger/upset/hurt someone else).
- Staying in a relationship you know you shouldn't be in (with someone who doesn't care about you/treats you badly/ignores you/is abusive/etc.) either because you can't see yourself deserving better or you're too worried about what other people will think to get out of what you know is a bad situation.
- Having a child, or thinking about having a child, for reasons that have nothing to do with your deep and honest desire to love and care for another human being.
- Fearing the future and not having any clear direction for your life, especially if your moods oscillate from one thing to another often and/or rapidly.
- Losing friendships with people you actually care about because they can't accept the way you act or the way you treat them or other people.

What The Therapist Says

There are a lot of concerns in this chapter that relate to the more common patterns found in codependence and relationship addiction. The first deals with our expectations of what we feel the world is supposed to be. Again, these views are deeply ingrained in our psyche and stem from the attitudes we have picked up and internalized while growing up. Most common sources for our world views are found in our parents' views and the culture we grow up in. The danger to these subconscious beliefs of how the world works is that it fills us with expectations as to who we "should" be. Oftentimes these ideals clash with how we feel about who we are or what we want out of life. In those of us battling with codependence our own wants and needs often take the back seat to what we believe other people expect of us.

While it is true that certain adherence to cultural expectations is sometimes required for personal survival and the functioning of society as a whole, there needs to be a healthy balance between self-actualization and social acceptance. In individuals dealing with relationship addiction external validation from friends, family, spouses, and "society" becomes the most important aspect of life. Even when a relationship addict realizes that what he or she is doing does not feel good that person will, more often than not, disregard such misgivings as long as possible before endangering the "wrath" of family and society as a whole. That can lead to people engaging and maintaining unhealthy, even abusive relationships for years or decades on end just because they fear the rejection of others or the failure of what they think is "expected" from them more than their discontent and pain.

For those who are lucky enough to possess adequate self-interest to break off an unhealthy relationship the situation still does not necessarily lead to immediate betterment. In people suffering from codependent attitudes the cause and solution to emotional distress are looked for in outside sources. If a relationship addict does not feel like the relationship he or she is in is fulfilling the emotional needs present then the person in question will see the reason for this problem in the partner rather than in the self. In turn, a solution to feeling this emptiness and lack of fulfillment is then sought in a change in external factors as well. A geographical move, a different life partner, new friends, these are just some of the "ways out" a codependent relationship addict will consider to escape his or her dilemma. Some flee into a career, others into the lives of their children; or they begin seeking a new, "better" partner to satisfy the emotional craving for self-validation.

I have to reiterate that this behavior is in no way limited to people of low intelligence or limited education. No matter how smart we are, we can only see the world through the set of attitudes and expectations we learned as children. If those views center on seeking self-worth from outside sources, than that is the only thing the codependent person will know how to do. These behaviors are so deeply ingrained that we hardly ever become conscious of them. And since there are so many different outside sources of "emotional feedback" to choose from, be they different "types" of partners, lifestyle, etc., individuals who hold these views can spend an entire lifetime chasing one potential source for self-validation after another without ever having to consider that this pattern itself might be the problem.

Do not misunderstand. Expectations as to what we feel is "right" or "wrong" in life are not a bad thing. Actually, without them we could never function at all, not as individuals or a society. But the level of how flexible or rigid our expectations are will determine how well we can adapt to the real world. People with extremely rigid expectations as to how life works and what is expected of them tend to suffer from a greater degree of obsession about pleasing others. "Getting things right" becomes more important than "feeling happy." As a result, individuals with such rigid belief structures tend to be perfectionists, equating their success in adhering to what they believe are society's norms to their own personal worth. Should they fall short of these expectations their sense of self takes a nosedive and they will frantically seek absolution by somehow "fixing" their shortcoming. Someone who suffered a "failed" marriage will either try to seek a better relationship to make up for the previous one or focus on success in a different aspect of life, maybe being a good parent or successful entrepreneur. All these solutions again deal with adhering to an external expectation, a measure of success that will ascertain approval from an external source.

A good indication as to whether a person puts too much emphasis on outside validation and norms is when communication patterns in the family exclude emotional content. If we grow up in an environment where feelings are not talked about in order to maintain certain appearances then the lesson we learn is that our inner mind is less important than the image we present to others. Or, if taken to a greater extreme, that outside opinions and validations are always more important than what we ourselves think and feel. Does anybody else notice the potential for disaster inherent in these concepts? If we have attained a subconscious world view where what we truly feel is subservient to what others think about us, what does that say about our chances of ever feeling content?

The answer is as simple as it is devastating: the chances of us achieving a permanent state of contentment while solely seeking self-worth through outside validation are almost exactly zero. Think about it. Few people will ever manage to please everybody they come into contact with. The chance of an individual having everybody they will ever meet like them are astronomical. One might have a greater possibility of winning the lottery, and more than once. But still many people live by just this kind of subconscious view, that worth and happiness are attained by satisfying outside expectations. If we could just please our parents, spouses, children, neighbors, society, and everyone else, or have them like us, then we could be happy. That is not a scenario that is likely to occur. But as you think back at the chapter you have just read, realize just how pervasive that innate world view is. With so many different ways to find outside sources of approval we can spend multiple lifetimes finding that "one" external source to make us happy without ever considering that this search is, in itself, the flaw that keeps us from being happy with ourselves.

Does that mean we are doomed to be locked into these patterns? Are we destined to be on a futile search for that obscure source of happiness and self-affirmation our entire lives? Of course not. Simply by realizing that what keeps us from being content is something that lies within us rather than a missing outside source is the first major step in breaking that useless old pattern of behavior. We can now turn inward and look at our own beliefs; those things we believe to be true about our own worth. Once we hone in on those core values, which can be done most easily by figuring out what situations make us feel bad about ourselves, we can then rationally question how reasonable these views truly are.

Is it reasonable to expect from us to always please our parents in whatever we do? Is it reasonable to assume that a "perfect person" will take away all our sorrows and emotional pains once we find him or her? Is it reasonable to assume we will be able to have everyone we meet like us? The more we think about these kinds of questions and allow ourselves to see how unreasonable our expectations of ourselves are, the more we can begin the process of changing these same expectations into views that are more accepting and self-affirming, without the need for outside validation.

Chapter 5: Marriage Number Three – Country Boy

I still vividly remember the first time I saw Alex. The first thing I noticed was his long, dark hair. Gorgeous. We made eye contact a few times, but he never came over to me. I wondered what was wrong with me that he wasn't interested. Just about the time I was looking at the bar and contemplating whether I'd need another beer to get the courage to go over to him, my friend elbowed me in the ribs and hissed under her breath that he was coming this way. He got within about six inches of me, veered off, and asked the girl at the table behind me if she wanted to dance. I was livid...and embarrassed because I had *thought* he was looking at me. What did she have that I didn't? I had an almost perverse urge to trip her when she walked past me, but that wouldn't have solved anything in the long run. I tried not to watch them dance, but I couldn't help myself. I was jealous...of a girl who I didn't know, dancing with a man who I had never met. How pathetic, but that was the story of my life. When I saw something I thought I wanted, for whatever reason, I wanted it right that moment...and thought I *deserved* it, just because it was something – or someone –I wanted. I had such a strong sense of entitlement, but yet I felt worthless, and the inner conflict was wearing me down.

I'm not even sure where the entitlement complex came from. I guess I thought I'd been 'made' to suffer enough from all the awful things other people had done to me. Now I should be able to put that all behind me and go on to the glory and great things that I'd surely be given. I wasn't working for any of these things. I wasn't even praying for them. I didn't even talk to God about it...I just worked at my menial job, and when I wasn't working I sat back and waited for wondrous and beautiful things to just flow into my life. Usually, I felt pretty good about it. I was sure my time was coming. Watching Alex and that other girl dance, though, my faith in the fact that I deserved better than what I had started to slip.

I started feeling really sorry for myself just about the time he appeared before me, hand outstretched, and asked me to dance. I thought about shunning him, because he'd hurt my feelings asking that other girl to dance first. He should apologize to me! But I was intrigued by him, and I was lonely and a little drunk, so I accepted. As we danced, he told me the girl sitting at the table behind me was a friend, and he figured he'd better dance with her before he asked me. He said he knew, once he asked me to dance, he was never going to want to dance with anyone else again. I could have melted into a puddle. What a romantic thing to say! You know that little part of your brain that points things out that you don't usually want to hear? The one that screams 'what a *line*!' when it hears something like that? It was clamoring desperately for my attention. Being the person I was, I stepped on it hard and went on with the dance.

We danced every slow dance that night, and stayed away from the fast ones. I didn't know how to line dance, and I still don't. When the bar closed we went to the beach and sat on a huge piece of driftwood and watched the waves by starlight. We talked about everything, and he finally got around to asking the question I was dreading – did I have children? I thought about lying, but knew it wasn't like I could just hide my little girl away, and I wasn't ashamed of *her*, after all, so I told the truth. He loved children, he said. He wanted to know all about her, and whether I wanted more in the future. I was astonished. He actually *wanted* a package deal – a woman *and* children. Perfect. I saw immediate stepfather potential, even though I didn't know him well enough to see anything. It's amazing how someone with a relationship or love addiction problem can see only what they want to see in someone else. We take only the good and we find excuses to overlook the bad, because we don't want to be alone again. I felt like I could make it work with this guy because he liked children, he was good looking, and he seemed like just a 'good ol' boy.' He wasn't overly intelligent and didn't have some kind of fantastic job but I saw potential, and I saw someone I could basically control. I had to be in charge, or there was just no way it would ever work out. I wasn't trusting my future to someone else – after all, I was doing such a good job of securing my future on my own. Yeah. Sure. I was at the stage of denying being in denial!

We dated for only five months. Both of us seemed hell-bent on marriage from the outset. I don't know if he was a relationship addict as well…it wasn't something I ever thought about at that time. I didn't even know what the term meant. All of the little aggravating things about Alex I just overlooked and ignored. I didn't want to see them. I just wanted to have someone in my life so I could feel important, and he would have to do. He asked me to marry him, and of course I accepted. How could I not? I was *somebody* when I was married. I conveniently seemed to forget I really didn't *like* being married, and I always felt trapped once I settled into the routine of it. It was the idea of *getting* married that I was in love with. It was exciting. Getting that ring, shopping for a dress, mailing out invitations. If I could just do all those things and then not actually *be* married that would be great, but it didn't work that way. I was counting on myself to do it right this time. I felt older and wiser, and Alex had been married once before.

Like me, Alex always blamed everything on everyone else. Nothing was ever his fault. His failed marriage was his ex-wife's fault, problems at his job were his supervisor's fault, etc. I felt bad for him, because he'd sustained a serious leg injury several years before in a freak accident, yet he worked doing framing and drywall every day, toughing it out even when it was very painful. I was proud he was that dedicated. I thought that kind of dedication would spill over into our marriage, which would be a great thing to have. My daughter seemed to like him well enough but she was a little bit uncertain, and that didn't improve over time like I thought it would. I don't think she was really old enough to understand why her father wasn't there anymore, and I didn't know how to explain that to a two-year-old in a way that would make sense to her. She seemed indifferent to whether Alex lived with us or not, and there were times she seemed to shy away from him. I figured it was just normal shyness at that age, and I did what I did so well with things I didn't want to see – I ignored it.

The day he gave me my engagement ring I had to hide my disappointment. Oh, it wasn't just the ring. I knew what I was getting with that. It came from a pawn shop, we had picked it out together, and we had been making payments on it. He'd moved in with me after only dating a couple of months, and we'd already combined most of our finances. Not that we had much money to combine. The day I got the ring one of the smaller stones fell out of it and I had to have it replaced. It wasn't the stone that ruined my day, though. It was the lack of any pomp and circumstance. We were getting *engaged.* Where was the down on one knee thing? Where were the flowers? Where was the poem he had written for me or the declarations of love I expected to hear? No. I got none of that. I showed him the ring I'd gotten fixed, and he took it out of the box and shoved it on my finger. He'd just come from work, and he was sitting on a kitchen chair, sweaty and dirty and stinky and exhausted. Yuck. Not the most romantic thing that had ever happened to me, by far. I took the ring anyway. I thought maybe he had something planned for later, or for the weekend. No. Wrong again. Another word was never said about it – until all the fights started. But first we had to have a wedding.

Neither one of us were big church-goers. I was baptized Christian thanks to my relationship with Tyler, and I believed in God, but I really didn't think much about Him in my day-to-day life, and that was about it. Alex was pretty much the same. He did know a minister through his mother, and we recruited that gentleman to perform the ceremony. We sent out a lot of invitations, and less than thirty people bothered to show up. The setting was an open-air amphitheater at a state park, and while it was beautiful, I was nervous and scared, feeling sick to my stomach. My daughter's father was invited, but didn't show up. I didn't really expect him to. He still had some animosity, and he was still hurt, and he hadn't bothered to be around very much since the divorce. He'd moved from my parents' house, and was making payments on a place about five miles from us. My father loaned him the down payment and co-signed the mortgage.

He did it not because he cared much about Tyler, but because he thought it was unfair to Karyn to be without her father. Without a place to live, he would have to go back to his parents' home, all the way across the country. Even though he lived close by I rarely saw him, and his daughter was steadily forgetting who he was. It was sad, but it was one of the few things that really *wasn't* my fault. I wasn't forcing him to stay away, and I never once told him he wasn't allowed to see his daughter. Ever. The court had granted him full visitation rights at all reasonable times and places, but he wasn't exercising them.

My daughter needed a father. Now, she was going to have a stepfather she could grow up around, and she'd adjust and we'd all be fine. That's what I told myself, over and over and over again, no matter what my gut feelings were. I'd been taught by my dad all my life to *think* about what I was doing, and so I ignored and suppressed those gut feelings. They weren't real. What was real was what your head told you, and what you could see and hear and touch – what was logical and tangible. That was all that mattered. I didn't know any better.

After Alex and I got through our wedding ceremony a limousine took us to his parents' house, where we had a reception in the backyard. It really was a nice time, but my most vivid memory of that day was of my daughter at the ceremony, hair pulled back in a ponytail and big green eyes fixed on me. My little flower girl, standing right next to me. She had one chubby fist wrapped around the material of my wedding dress, pointing at it with her other hand. I looked down to see a small, harmless, winged insect. 'Mommy!' she stage-whispered, loud enough for everyone to hear, 'There's a *bug* on your dress!' I just winked at her and told her it was OK, listening to the gentle laughter of the wedding party and assembled guests. She was not quite three years old yet, and she thought this was a big production she was involved in. She didn't know just what to make of it, but all three of us seemed to be happy that day. Third time's a charm, right?

Wrong. So wrong…and going more and more wrong with each passing day. My first serious clue about that was when my grandmother died. She'd been in a nursing home up in the north, suffering from Alzheimer's disease for several years. I remember visiting her when we lived nearby, and she'd even lived with us for a while before the disease got too bad for us to take care of her, but I never really knew her well. I tried to avoid her. I was young and she was just an old woman who I thought I had nothing in common with, and I didn't feel comfortable around her. She was always accusing me of stealing her things. I didn't really understand that it was just the disease talking, and that she didn't know what she was saying. I thought she hated me. I guess I really didn't like her that much, either. I didn't know how to. Overall, I wasn't a very nice person. I was raised with the idea that I should look out for myself, because the rest of the world wasn't going to, but I took that idea just a little bit too far, and I was too caught up in my own existential angst to even see it – like so much of society seems to be today.

My mother and I had been shopping, and we got back and my father walked out to meet us. He told my mom that the nursing home had called just a few minutes ago, and that her mother had died. 'I'm sorry,' he muttered awkwardly, and he patted her shoulder a couple of times and went back in the house, leaving her standing in the yard crying, and leaving me to comfort her. Here came another fourteen-hour trip! We left that night and I drove. We took mom's car because it was bigger, and I left Alex my car. My beautiful little Karyn had to stay behind. It was too much of a trip to try to take a very young child, and she wouldn't understand what was going on anyway. She refused to stay with Alex, becoming scared when I said anything about it. She wanted to stay with her grandpa, and she clung to him. She ended up sleeping on the love seat at my mom and dad's house while we were gone. My father slept on the couch, to be nearby if she woke in the night and was scared. It should have bothered me that she didn't want to stay alone in the house with Alex. It should have been a huge red flag. I'd like to think that, if I hadn't been so wrapped up in trying to comfort my mother and get us safely to her mother's funeral, I would have noticed it and questioned it, but I don't honestly know whether it would have made any difference. I just don't know. That's what happens when you only see what you want to see. I chalked it up to the fact that she didn't know Alex that well yet and was upset I was leaving, and I went on with my life.

Once we got back home from the funeral, life settled into a more normal routine. I stayed home with my daughter, and Alex worked his framing and drywall job. We bought a German Shepherd mix puppy from a guy selling them at the flea market. Eventually, I took a job at a convenience store and my parents watched my daughter when I had to work. Tyler was basically non-existent. Alex and I had little money, but we did all right. We were able to pay our bills and buy food and cigarettes, but that was about all we could safely do. We started to use credit cards to buy some things, and the bills began to pile up. We couldn't pay them off, but we managed to make the minimum payments. Because paying on time gave us a decent credit rating we got other credit cards, and soon we had three or four with several thousand dollars worth of credit available on each one. We maxed them out, and then Alex started to want more things. We didn't have the money, and he wanted to know what I was spending it on. Never mind the three hundred dollars he had spent for the old truck that he was going to fix up that still sat, rusting, in our yard. Never mind all the cigarettes he smoked or the beer he drank or the tools he needed for work or the things he was buying and bringing home to 'fix up' the house or the deck that we built out back. Never mind the baby bunnies and rats he had to buy to feed the three snakes he'd brought with him, or the special food for his iguana.

What was *I* spending *our* money on? Food. Gasoline. Bathroom tissue. Things we needed. I was still being accused of being wasteful, though, and I got tired of that very quickly. As if our money problems weren't big enough, Alex's leg injury got so bad that he had to have surgery. That meant at least six weeks off work, with no weight on his leg at all. I had to do everything – pay all the bills off my income, run the household, get him anything he needed, and take care of my daughter. The doctor told him to forget about going back to any kind of construction work at all. He should take up a different profession. With only a high school education, what was he supposed to do? Go back to school, of course. I had to pay for that, too.

He enrolled at the local community college to be a mechanic. He took the transmission in his own, personal truck apart because it was acting up, and he never could get it back together right. My parents paid to have the truck towed to a local garage and fixed. Naturally, it cost more because Alex had 'fixed' it first. My dad said the money was a loan, but it never got paid back. Every time I had another marriage, my parents wrote off the debt I had racked up to them as a wedding gift to me. One marriage got me out of over twenty thousand dollars, but I can't even remember any more which marriage that was. The write-off was something I had started to take for granted by the third or fourth time, anyway.

The mechanic thing didn't work out very well. Alex never could get the hang of it. When his leg healed he went back to construction work instead. All of his tuition money might as well have gone straight in the garbage. We were paying for the house, the car, the truck, and about four credit cards each month, plus our regular household bills…and we were rapidly losing ground. Having only one or two hundred dollars in the bank as a running balance was not uncommon, and things weren't getting any better. That wasn't the only problem. The other problem was the shower. Alex seemed to have forgotten what it was for. He was always clean and smelled nice when we were dating. Once that ring was on my finger, I guess he just assumed soap was no longer necessary. Have you ever wanted to have sex with someone who works out in the heat all day and doesn't shower for a week or so? I certainly didn't. It made me gag just to think about it, and he accused me of not meeting his needs. He stunk so badly I couldn't stand to touch him. His teeth were turning brown from smoking so much and never brushing them, and he had gained about twenty-five pounds. His own mother even commented on it, so I know it wasn't just me.

I don't think I'm beautiful. I think I'm average-looking. Not ugly, certainly, but not all that pretty, either. I'm just a normal person. But my teeth are white because I brush them and take care of them, and my hair is clean and my clothes are clean and I know what a shower is for. I'm not overweight, and I try to take care of myself. That's all I ask of others who share my life. Just take care of yourself. It's common courtesy to stay clean and to take a shower if you get sweaty. I thought it was a normal thing that everyone did. Instead, I became the 'frigid wife' who wouldn't give him what he needed. He wanted his coffee ready in the morning and his lunch packed, we ate dinner with my parents, and he wanted me to fulfill my 'wifely duties' each night, no matter how strange his requests and ideas became.

When I refused I was badgered and sneered at. When I complied I had to force down the nausea. I tried to talk to him, what I believed to be openly and honestly, about the problems we were having. He made everything out to be my fault, and I in turn made everything out to be his fault. There was no agreement. He thought I was a little 'ice princess' who thought I was too good for him, and I thought he was gross and disgusting.

Some of the most vivid memories I have of him involve him sticking his filthy, stinking feet under my nose because he thought it was funny, and of the night he threw all three of my cats outside during a violent hailstorm because one of them had broken some little trinket he had bought me, and that I didn't really like that much anyway. I yelled at him for that, and it escalated into a huge fight. He asked whether I would choose the cats over him, because that was what it sounded like. I didn't say a word, and I guess my silence made it clear to him. He shut his mouth, let the cats back in, and went to bed without another word. In the morning, he acted like nothing had ever happened. Overall, the same patterns continually showed up on the doorstep of our marriage – where is all the money going? Why are you denying me sex? Why are your parents always in our business? Why doesn't your daughter call me daddy? Doesn't she love me? Don't *you* love me?

Those were the biggest issues – my daughter and my parents. My parents were too involved, my daughter wasn't involved enough. Never mind the fact that my parents were always helping us out, lending us money if we needed it, and letting Alex use the barn they had and all the tools. Never mind that my daughter was getting the creeps because her stepdaddy was a little too affectionate and he was unclean and reeked of smoke and sweat. I didn't think then, and I still don't think now, that a stepfather should kiss a female child on the mouth or pat her on the butt but he did both, quite frequently. He would do it before bed, when she got back from being at grandma and grandpa's house, or just when she was walking by. He spent a lot of time looking at her, calling her sweetheart, stroking her hair, commenting on how pretty she was. He kept insisting it was harmless, and he told me a huge sob-story about his ex-wife, and how she was pregnant and lost his baby, and he was heartbroken. He just wanted a child to love. In fact, he wanted *children* to love. He wanted us to have a child together. I agreed. What the hell was I thinking? I don't know. Why any people who got along like we did would try to bring a child into the world, I can't explain. Why any mother who didn't trust her new husband with her young daughter would try to have a child with him I also

124

can't explain. That's the kind of blindness that relationship and love addiction bring to a person.

We stopped using protection and he started taking a little better care of himself, brushing his teeth more often and staying marginally cleaner, hoping to entice me. I tried, in an effort of reconciliation, to make myself more available to him more often. Soon after, I suspected I was pregnant, but I didn't say anything to him about it. Even though I had agreed to it initially, now that it might be a reality I felt sort of sick about it. About three weeks later my period finally came, late, but it wasn't like anything I normally experienced. I felt sick, shaky, and feverish, and I had extreme cramping accompanied by clots. I had lost the baby, I assumed. I didn't even go to the doctor to find out if that's what really happened. I was secretly glad, and that made me feel awful for the sake of the little life that might have been. Maybe this was my punishment for the fact that I almost aborted Karyn? I tried to find more reasons to avoid sex with Alex as much as possible after that, because I didn't want to go through that again, and I realized that I really didn't want anything to do with mothering his child. He wasn't going to change, and I sure wasn't impressed with him the way he was.

When I told him I'd changed my mind and no longer wanted to have a baby he was angry, and since he didn't want to go back to using protection – using the standard male excuse that it didn't feel as good – we basically reached an impasse where marital relations were concerned. I was slowly coming to my senses about his abuse, as well. Too many people think that abuse only means that a person hits you. That's what I always thought. It can mean that, sure, but it can also mean verbal abuse, and that was his specialty. He badgered me so badly for sex one night that I was sobbing, literally crying uncontrollably, as I gave in. He stopped, pushed me away, and sneered.

"You can put your clothes back on," he said, and he rolled over, away from me, muttering "God, I can't even *guilt* you into it." That was what our marriage had been reduced to.

My self-esteem was at its lowest point by then. He had been verbally abusing me nearly the entire time we had been married, but I had tried to pass it off as 'just the way he talked.' I knew I wasn't stupid, but I was starting to feel like I was. He had beaten me down so far that I wasn't sure how to get back up again. I felt worthless as a wife, worthless as a woman, and worthless as a person. It was around that time that Maximillian, who had moved to my area based on a job offer, decided to look me up. He never was one to hold a grudge, and he was always so forgiving of everyone. He wasn't still angry with me for ending our long-distance love affair the way I did, before it ever really got started. He just pulled up in my driveway one day, not knowing I'd gotten married again. I ran out and threw my arms around him and picked him up off the ground...and then I realized that Alex had followed me outside and was standing behind me. I introduced them, although I hated to. Maximillian sure looked good. I couldn't believe I had let him go and had ended up with a trashy abuser who never took care of himself. What had I been thinking? I felt like I was nothing but trailer trash now, and I couldn't imagine how anyone as classy and put-together as Max could ever want anything to do with me again. Maybe someday...but that was only wishful thinking.

I had become someone who I never wanted to be. A person who was trashy, a person who was the 'little woman' who did what her husband said, a person who was only ever going to squeak by with a meager existence instead of enjoying everything that life had to offer. I don't look down on people who choose to live in trailers, or who don't have the choice, and I don't look down on women who choose to follow their husband's lead if that's what truly makes them happy. I'm not that judgmental. But at that time in my life I suffered from the belief that I wasn't good enough, so I associated it with my circumstances. I'd gone from thinking I deserved better than what I'd been through to feeling like I didn't deserve anything good. I still wished for something better, though. I still dreamt of it. If I had a nice house and a good husband I'd be happy, right? I doubt it would have made a difference, but I thought it would. I insisted on looking for outside problems and faults, instead of looking on the inside of myself to see what was missing. People just didn't do that back then, or if they did I hadn't been told about it. Another dilemma of growing up with such a sheltered existence. I wasn't exposed to many bad things as a child, but I wasn't exposed to things that could help me, either. I wasn't exposed to anything. When life caught up with me I was exposed to so many things all at once I was overloaded and didn't know where to turn. I couldn't focus.

After Max left, I couldn't stop thinking about him. Alex saw that, I think, but I kept insisting it didn't matter, and that it was a long time ago. When I was alone I daydreamed about what kind of life I might have been able to have with Maximillian. When I was around Alex I tried to pretend to be happy but the bills just got worse, and so did the abuse. I was stupid. I couldn't cook. I was letting myself go. I didn't smile enough. Why wasn't I more friendly? Why was I tired when we went to bed at night? I dreaded the nighttime, because I knew we were going to fight about our 'marital relations' – or lack thereof. I was becoming increasingly more nervous during the evening hours. He finally stopped asking for sex at all, which actually made me more nervous. Was he getting it somewhere else? He said he wasn't, but he also said quite honestly that he would *have to* eventually, because *men* have *needs*, and if I wouldn't fulfill them some woman would be required to. He wasn't interested in getting divorced, he was just interested in having some sex on the side. I was horrified. What a terrible thing to say. Of course, I wasn't the model wife, either.

I kicked him out twice over the next year, but we were always reconciled. Him because he didn't want to be 'defeated' by a woman and kept trying to win me back, only to go right back to the same old thing within a few days of moving back in. Me out of sheer ignorance, I guess. I didn't want to be alone, but I didn't want Alex, either…and I didn't want to be a failure again. I was weak. What I wanted most of all was for my parents to say I should leave him. Then I would know they approved and I could go ahead and do it, but of course they weren't going to say that. Parents – most parents – don't council their children to leave their marriages, especially when they themselves have been married for many years and have made it work no matter what. So I was still stuck, and thinking about how miserable I was and how life was so unfair for me. I went back and forth between being angry and thinking I deserved better and being depressed and thinking I deserved just what I had at that moment – that was all that was there for me in this life. I thought about suicide.

After all, I owned a gun. It would be easy, and quick. It would probably be painless, too, if I did it right. Just here one second and gone the next. In the end, I couldn't do that to Karyn. She saved me, more than once, even though she never knew it. How ironically beautiful that a life I had almost ended helped me to save my own.

On a Saturday in May, Alex wanted me to come up back to the barn with him and help him work on a vehicle. I figured I might as well…at least it was a nice day outside, and it was later in the afternoon, so it wouldn't be an all-day event. I hadn't felt that well all day. I was vaguely nervous about something I couldn't put my finger on, and I kept thinking about my dad. I should go to see him. I didn't really want to make the drive. It was almost thirty minutes. It bothered me all day. Karyn was with my mom, and my dad was at the flea market, where he had a booth and sold odds and ends. We hadn't been working long when my dad's truck came pulling in, a little more slowly than usual. I didn't think much of it as he made his way to my parents' house, carrying his lunch box. He was in his early sixties, and he was still pretty spry. I didn't think much about his age.

A few short minutes later my mother was yelling at us and waving frantically from the front porch. I thought she was just waving until I realized she was making those universal 'come here' motions. I ran to her and she told me my dad thought he had had a stroke. It took him what seemed like forever to convey that to her – he could barely speak. The words were all in his head, but what he needed to get them from there to his mouth wasn't working right any more. Stubborn as he was (and still is), he didn't even want to go to the hospital, but we convinced him to at least go and have his blood pressure checked. They kept him three days. He couldn't speak more than a few words, and he was pissed about having to stay in that sterile white room with his butt hanging out of a gown while people poked and prodded him. He'd had a headache for four days and hadn't told anyone, and once he had his stroke at around nine in the morning, he stayed at the flea market all day making sales even though he couldn't talk, and then he packed up his things all by himself and drove himself home. That basically says everything that anyone would ever need to know about my dad.

I was wracked with guilt. All that day I'd felt as though I should go see him, but I didn't because I didn't feel like I wanted to make the drive. I was lazy. I could have done something. Helped him pack. Called 911. Driven him to the hospital. Been his voice. Just sat there and told him it would be all right; taken care of *him* for once. Something. In the end, we were all blessed. He came home on a Wednesday, was put on some low-dose medication, and gained back his speech. He went back to the flea market the next weekend. Stubborn, and dedicated. I remember my daughter running up to me a few weeks later, after being left alone in grandpa's care for the first time since the stroke. She was carrying a book.

"Come here, mommy," she said. "Look how well grandpa reads!"

I burst into tears.

Occasionally my dad speaks more slowly than he used to, and sometimes a word doesn't come out quite right, but if you didn't know him before, you'd never notice it. I always notice it, but then, I still feel guilty, too. I shouldn't. I doubt very seriously my dad is still thinking about it, but I always will.

We followed my parents the day it happened. My mother drove my dad to the hospital, with Alex and Karyn and I lagging behind in our car. Alex almost didn't go. His friend was supposed to come over, and he didn't want to leave. It would be rude. I told him if he didn't get in the car, he wasn't to be there when I got back. This was my *dad.* Alex's mother had experienced several heart attacks and other health-crisis episodes since we'd met, and I was always there. Always. It didn't matter what else was going on. It didn't matter what time it was. And this was what I got for that? The cruelty and indifference he had was almost unbelievable to me. It was just one more straw on the camel's back. It wasn't the one that broke it, but it was getting dangerously close, and it only made the problems we already had worsen and grow stronger. It made me dislike him more, which made me bitchy and short-tempered around him, which made him dislike me more. What a life.

Shortly after that, as if my stress levels weren't high enough already, my parents ended up spending thousands of dollars to help me settle a lawsuit out of court. Every time Tyler came by, his daughter would cry and scream. She didn't want to go with him. He came by so infrequently she didn't know who he was any more. He would always back down and leave her there with me and then he sued me, saying I was denying him his rights and teaching her that Alex was her father. It caused a serious amount of tension for a long period of time, and it took us many months to settle the issue. Eventually, he dropped the suit and we signed a mediation agreement that granted him the same damn rights he already had. A pointless waste of time and money on both sides.

The first day he came to pick Karyn up after the agreement was signed by the judge, I had to physically pry her from me and force her into his car, and she screamed like crazy. She was terrified, but he put her through it anyway. She was too young to understand that mommy could go to jail if little Karyn didn't get in the car and go with her daddy. It was incredibly heart-wrenching, and I wasn't sure how I was going to stand it. I really felt like my heart might actually break. I cried as he drove away with her. To his credit, he did call me later so I could hear the silence – she had stopped screaming. That pattern of him showing up infrequently and her crying and not wanting to go with him continued throughout her younger years. Later, it turned from crying into a sense of resignation, then to a deep and serious loathing, and finally to a grudging indifference.

It was just another problem that Alex and I had to deal with, and he wasn't always very graceful in his way of handling it. If he hadn't been so insistent about Karyn calling him 'daddy' and I hadn't been willing to let myself be bullied into it, the whole lawsuit issue might never have happened. Either way, it didn't reflect very well on Tyler or on Alex, or on me, really. In an effort to make himself look good (and get out of the house more), Alex joined up with our local volunteer fire department. After a few weeks I wanted to join it, too. I didn't like him having new friends, because I couldn't control what he did around them, and it upset me. Plus, I really didn't have any friends to speak of, and I didn't want to look bad to others. I was suspicious…who knows what he was saying to these people about me and our relationship? I didn't trust him. I always thought people were talking about me behind my back. It was probably a throwback to the harassment I'd suffered in school, but wherever it came from, it wasn't going away. So I joined, too. I should have known it wasn't the place for me. They asked me why I wanted to join. I said I wanted to help people. They laughed like I'd made a great joke, but they found me a uniform and a pager and signed me up. I looked like a little girl playing dress-up in all that big, heavy gear. But I took it home and waited eagerly to go on my first call. I thought I was cool. Here was a place where I could make a difference. I *mattered*.

I soon found out it was mostly older people who needed medical help that, despite the fact that they had dialed 911, was really of the non-urgent variety – what the other volunteers called 'frequent flyers' – instead of the more exciting calls I'd been expecting. I wanted to save someone from a burning building, or at least be there so I could get some of the credit. I finally got to go on a real call, only to have it cut short because it was actually in another jurisdiction and they didn't need our help. I was almost in tears, riding in that giant fire truck with the siren wailing away and all the lights flashing. It was overwhelming and exciting. I felt so important, like I could do so much good for the world…like I had a purpose. We got back to the station just in time for me to go and pick up Alex from his job. After I collected him and we were heading home I was just driving along, drinking a soda and listening to the radio, when I was suddenly overwhelmed with terror. My heart was pounding, my hands were shaking, I was sweating, and I was completely engulfed with fear. I'd never experienced anything like it. I wanted to bolt from the car and curl up into a ball, both at the same time. I did neither. I just kept driving. We passed a hospital, and I had to fight the urge not to turn into the parking lot, run to the emergency room, and beg them to save me, but I made it home. I had no idea what in the world was happening.

Over the next few days I kept feeling like that, on and off. It never completely went away, and I never felt 'well.' I spent most of my time on the couch, huddled in a blanket. I thought maybe I had the flu. I didn't play with my daughter, I didn't work, and I didn't do much of anything. I couldn't eat, and I lost weight. On my already slender frame that wasn't a good idea, and I got very weak. I was cold and then hot, sick to my stomach, and there was a lump in my throat. My hands wouldn't stop shaking. My heart raced, and I had trouble sleeping. Maybe I was dying? My daughter was so young…would she even remember me? Alex was sympathetic for a couple of days. After that, he insisted there was nothing wrong with me. If I hadn't died by now I must be fine, right? I went to the only doctor in my area that public assistance would pay for and told him my symptoms. I asked him if it could have anything to do with my prolapsed mitral valve. He said no, and he did an EKG, examined me, and told me that, if I felt like that again, I was probably having a heart attack and should go to the hospital. I was twenty-four. What were my heart attack odds? And what about the 'heart attack' I was having right then? But I believed him. I went home feeling worse, and sure that I was dying. My poor little daughter would never know me. I'd die as Alex's wife, too, and I was beginning to loathe Alex. There was no sympathy, and no one seemed that concerned.

For the first time in my adult life, I really, seriously felt like my parents let me down. It would've been nice if they would've spent some of their money to see if I really *was* dying, but they didn't. They just told me I was fine. I had good days and bad days, and then my heart started skipping beats, and I became terrified all the time again; convinced this was the end. My daughter was four. When a few weeks went by and I was still alive, I decided I needed to figure out what was wrong on my own. No one else was apparently going to do it for me. Again, I felt put-upon, like I was always being required to do everything…even though I knew that really wasn't the case. I always had to have an excuse and it always had to be someone else's fault – but this time I feared I really was seriously sick. I kept thinking about what the doctor had said, but I didn't go to the emergency room the next time I felt that way, and I didn't die. Since it looked like I was going to survive I went to the library, shaking hands, skipping heart, and all.

I took a deep breath and used the library computer to search their records for mitral valve prolapse and my search returned some books, one of which gave me a tremendous amount of insight when I flipped through it. I checked it out, took it home, and read it from cover to cover. Finally, I understood at least a part of what was wrong with me. I think, if the book had belonged to me instead of the library, I would have carried it down to the doctor who 'diagnosed' me and cheerfully shoved it right up his ass, so he could read it at his leisure. Instead, I settled for trying to explain to Alex what was wrong, so he could help me feel better. He never read the book. He wasn't interested in anything other than me 'acting right' again, so I could go back to doing what I was 'supposed' to do. My parents never read the book, either. When I told my father what I found out he said "Oh. Good," and went back to watching television. He didn't want to deal with anything that was outside his comfort zone – or maybe he just didn't know how to.

What I'd had was a panic attack, brought on by a complex but non-life-threatening issue called 'mitral valve prolapse syndrome,' and over the next few weeks I learned how to avoid many of the attacks and understand the ones I did have. I experimented. For several days I drank water and avoided caffeine, and I felt better. Then I ate a candy bar and drank a cappuccino. It wasn't twenty minutes before my heart was skipping like crazy, my chest hurt, I couldn't breathe well and my hands were shaking. That told me everything I needed to know about what to do and not to do, but even then it didn't always work. The panic attacks didn't go away overnight, either, and Alex couldn't understand why I wasn't 'fixed.' I still had a lot of symptoms, and I had to change my eating habits and make some other modifications so I could feel better as much as possible. I even went back to work to make some more money for the household, but he complained that I wasn't home enough at night, so I quit. I couldn't please him, no matter what I did. I couldn't please myself, either. Something was always wrong, either physically, mentally, or both.

We even stopped going fishing together, and that was something we'd done almost every weekend once we started dating, and it had continued into our married life. We usually took Karyn, who loved going on another "fishin' mission." Sometimes I still miss the fishing…the cool nights, the salt breeze, standing on the edge of the dock throwing the cast net, just seeing what kinds of things we could bring in. For a while we even sold to bait shops for extra money, and we ate some of the fish we caught and froze our own bait so we spent less money, both for food and for fishing. It helped us keep our heads above water financially, and once the fighting and unhappiness escalated to the point that the fishing stopped, the bills only got worse. We lived in the same house, but we weren't together. We said very little to one another. After a few weeks of this, I noticed he was getting up earlier and earlier to go to work. I wasn't sure why, other than I figured he was checking his email.

My parents had given us a used computer, and we had dial-up service for the Internet. We'd only had it for a couple of months, maybe, but we used it a lot. For some reason I started paying attention to Alex's morning routine. Some little sixth sense – the one I kept trying to ignore – kept waking me up early to make me more aware of it. He was getting up about thirty to forty-five minutes before he'd need to in order to get ready and get to work on time, which put his waking time at around four-thirty in the morning. Who wants to get up that early if they don't have to? And why would it take that long to check email? Dial up was slow, but it wasn't *that* slow.

I asked, but he shrugged it off, saying he didn't like to rush in the morning, so I let it go. About three weeks later I got one of those 'psychic flash' thoughts…the kind that you *know* you didn't actually think, but they're suddenly just there. Like somebody else spoke right into your head. I'd had them quite a lot throughout my childhood, but they made me nervous and I did my best to repress them, along with an abundance of other strangeness that seemed to repeatedly happen to me. I didn't want to be 'different' in some other way, too; I got picked on enough without that. They went along with those 'gut feelings' my father seemed to think were a waste of time. I wanted to please him so badly I blocked out my 'spiritual side' and stuck to good old fashioned logic – which didn't seem to be serving me well.

This thought was about the computer and Alex, and it basically said 'he's looking at porn, not checking his email.' Was he? Really? Well…maybe. There *had* been the issue with the previous pornography problem. A few months previously I'd found a surprisingly large collection of pornographic videotapes hidden under one of the cages he kept his snakes in. He insisted they belonged to a friend, and he was just keeping them, because the friend wanted him to watch them and he didn't want to be rude. The friend lived just down the street, so I accompanied him to take the tapes back. When he handed them over and said 'here are those tapes you loaned me,' I could almost hear him saying 'wink, wink...I'll come back and get them from you later.' If he got them back he hid them better, because I never found them again – and I *did* look. I'd lived such a sheltered life throughout most of my existence that I'd seen very little pornography. I saw the Playboy channel once or twice with my cousin when his mother wasn't home, and I'd seen some 'dirty magazines' in high school, but that was the extent of my pornography experience. I really was clueless about how a person even *found* porn on the Internet, and I'd certainly never seen any, nor did I want to.

The thought kept nagging me...running over and over in my head. I finally sat down at the computer, got on the Internet, and went to the 'help/live chat' feature my service provider offered. I told the anonymous person on the other end I thought someone was using my computer to view pornography, and I wanted to know how to find out. I was given some simple steps to follow, and I was soon staring at a history folder for the last week. In seven days Alex had viewed pornographic sites over five hundred and thirty times! All of it was in the morning, while he was 'checking his email.' I copied down some of the sites, and I went to them...not all of them were 'standard' Playboy-type sites with naked women. There were bondage sites...and there were some sites where the participants definitely didn't look old enough to be doing what they were doing. Were they really underage, or did they just look it? Was it child porn? I wasn't sure, and couldn't really tell, but I had my suspicions – and he was being so affectionate with my precious little girl!

I was nauseated, and the room was spinning. I thought for a few minutes I might pass out. No. No, no, no. He *had* to go. I couldn't tolerate this, and I couldn't risk her. She already shied away from him more and more, and now I was terrified there might be a reason for that. Had he done something to her, or did she just sense something wasn't right? What was I going to do? I had no job, and I had no money. I also had to find a way to convince my parents that Alex shouldn't be around their granddaughter. It was an easy thing to do where my mom was concerned. I showed her the sites, and she was just as repulsed by the whole thing as I was. She tried to talk to my dad. *I* tried to talk to my dad. His answer was to shrug it off and say a lot of guys like to look at Playboy and things like that. I told him again that wasn't what this was. I even gave him specifics, but he clammed up and wouldn't talk about it anymore. I offered to show him. He looked at me like I'd sprouted a second head. I had to find a different way, because I couldn't bear to take the blame for another failed marriage but I couldn't let my daughter be endangered, especially when she was just starting to grow up and wasn't yet capable of defending herself.

I confronted Alex when he got home. He played dumb for as long as he could, and then he tried to turn the whole thing around to be my fault. If I just gave him what he needed, he wouldn't have to do this. He had to get some excitement *somewhere*. Needless to say, there was a huge fight involved that went on for hours. I didn't throw him out, because I thought if I did I would be blamed by my father, and I didn't want that. I couldn't take it, and I had quite a few days of depression. The panic attacks that had subsided came back again, and I kept struggling with symptoms. The mitral valve prolapse syndrome, or 'dysautonomia' meant that my nervous system was overly sensitive and didn't always work right. Even though I knew it wasn't dangerous it sure felt like it was, and it made me feel lousy a lot of the time, especially when I was under stress. Having all these issues with Alex just made it worse. I couldn't seem to calm down long enough for my high-strung nervous system to reset itself to a more normal mode. Why did I keep choosing these troublesome men? I tried to tell myself it wasn't me. It wasn't my fault. It was just that they were deceitful, and they didn't show me who they truly were until after the wedding, at which point I was already stuck. If truth be told, it wasn't like there weren't any signs beforehand. It was that I didn't bother to look for them and didn't want to see them, even when they were right in front of me.

I decided to resort to the only other thing I knew to do – I would act so horribly that Alex would leave on his own, thus making it 'his fault' in my father's eyes, and keeping me from taking the blame. Yes, it was a lousy thing to do. I should have just owned up and said I'd made a mistake, and I should have just filed for divorce. It was my life, and it wasn't up to my parents. I couldn't see that, because I was still too convinced my parents wouldn't love me if I screwed up another marriage. Actually, that's not quite true. I knew my mother was behind me because of the porn I had found on the computer. I thought my *dad* wouldn't love me anymore. How can you keep loving a screw-up kid that always disappoints you and never does anything right? I couldn't keep a husband, apparently, and if my dad stopped loving me then I would feel like I was just worthless in the eyes of all men. In reality that was silly. I had cousins and an uncle who loved me...but we weren't close, and I didn't have the terror of displeasing them like I did with my father. I remember my dad telling me several times when I was a child that he was very disappointed in me when I had done something wrong. I never wanted to hear him say those words again. It was like a knife to my heart.

Since I didn't have a job I stayed home with my daughter all day, and I smoked cigarettes and read books and played on the Internet. I didn't even feel much like playing with her, and she often went to my parents' house to play with them, while I sat alone and tried not to think about anything. I was depressed, and I was losing weight again. Given the choice, I probably wouldn't have bothered to get out of bed in the morning. Some days, I was determined to fix this. Other days I just wanted to die, yet I was terrified of the idea as well. I tried to hoard every spare penny I could, so I would have a few hundred dollars when Alex was gone. That seemed like a lot of money to me then. I offered him nothing, just going through the motions of being a wife. I picked fights, I sighed theatrically every time I had to do something, and I started sleeping in Karyn's room with her. I did that for two reasons: I knew that Alex wouldn't like it because he wouldn't get sex, and I wanted to keep my little girl safe from harm, in case he wanted to try out something he saw on the Internet. I wasn't going to let her be the victim of that if I could avoid it. I might not have been a nice person, and I might not have done things right in a lot of ways, but I cared about my daughter, and I wanted to protect her...but I hated the idea that she would be without a stepfather.

On a stormy night a couple months later I was sitting on the couch, and Alex started pacing the floor. Karyn was asleep in her room. I asked him to stop, because he kept walking back and forth in front of the TV, and I couldn't see the program I was watching. My parents had given us an expensive satellite system, and I loved watching all the things I could never find on the three channels we got when I was a kid. Of course it was another bill to pay, but I was trying not to think about that. Alex started in on me as to why I was such a bitch. I just shrugged, pretending to watch TV while he got louder and louder. When he didn't get a reaction, he stomped into the bedroom and packed a bag. He came back out, went to the front door, and looked back at me, asking if I even cared he was leaving. I just gazed calmly back.

"I hope you die a lonely old bitch!" he said, and he walked out and slammed the door.

I cried from both relief and heartache for a long time after he was gone, hugging the Shepherd puppy that we had bought at the flea market, who had by then turned into a beautiful and tender-hearted dog who didn't seem to think I deserved the pain I was dealing with. She sat on the couch beside me, occasionally pressing her soft nose against my cheek as I balled my fists into her fur and sobbed. She never once yelped or tried to get away, although I'm sure I probably pulled her hair. She understood. When I just couldn't cry any more I went to bed, alone, and actually slept well for the first time in months.

In the morning my mom came by to check on me because she didn't see Alex's truck and it wasn't a workday for him. When I saw her coming I sat on the couch, head in my hands. I had to have the theatrics right, even for her. If I played the game properly, both of my parents would blame Alex and I would be comforted by them. I could feel safe again. I told my mom he had left me – just walked out and left me, and I told her what his last words to me had been. That much, at least, was true. He *had* walked out and left me. Of course, I didn't mention the way I'd been treating him lately. I gave the same story to my father that night. He didn't really seem that angry, but a week later when he found a bunch of his tools missing from the barn he was much more annoyed. I knew then that Alex wouldn't be forgiven, and I was off the hook regarding the blame game. I was good at being deceitful, and I was good at getting what I wanted, with the exception of decent men and money.

I wasn't off the hook regarding the bills, though. After Alex showed up and collected all his things (asking me about taking Karyn to the park, just him and her, which I flatly refused), I filed for divorce and went looking for a job. I finally found a minimum wage clerical job in a neighboring city almost an hour away. That was the best I could do, given that I didn't have a steady work history and had never finished even my two-year college degree, dropping out when I was pregnant with Karyn because I had so much morning sickness I couldn't function well. The girl I shared the office with was really nice. She even bought me lunch almost every day and bought presents for my daughter that year for Christmas...but while I appreciated it what I really needed was a raise, and that wasn't going to happen. I wanted to be paid what she was paid. She did less work than me and made twice as much money, but she was the boss' daughter.

She tried to fix me up with everyone she could find, which was fine because I was lonely. After all the bad experiences I'd had you would've thought I would've been gun-shy, but I wasn't. I was too desperate to belong to someone again. Without at least a steady boyfriend I wasn't anyone but me, and that wasn't very impressive at all. Who was I to think I was somebody? She introduced me to a man who was a manager at a large local company. An important man within the community. I was impressed, because he was very attractive and much older than me. I saw a chance at having a 'sugar daddy,' but I didn't know him all that well. I finally got tired of dancing around the issue, so I called him and invited him out for a beer. He accepted, and we met at a bar near his house. I was trying to show off and match him beer for beer, and I got pretty drunk pretty fast. He invited me to come to his house for a while and sleep it off. I said no. He was essentially a stranger. He gave me a big speech about how he would never take advantage of someone who had been drinking. What kind of a person did I think he was? I went to his house, and he raped me. Aggressively. To the point that I was still crying as I fished broken pieces of condom from inside my body the following day.

As horrified and disgusted as I was I didn't tell anyone, and I didn't report it. I blocked it out, locked it away, and told myself it had been consensual – even though I knew it hadn't been. I even saw him a few more times, trying to convince myself that I'd wanted the sex and we could have a relationship, but there was no more sex involved in those meetings. He was just a horny old man who couldn't seem to keep his hands out of my pants when I was around him, so I stopped seeing him and I stopped taking his calls. I was relieved when he finally just took the hint and went away, but I still felt horrible. I felt I'd deserved it. After all, I was the lonely girl who got drunk with a stranger and then went to his house. I trusted him. How stupid was that? I guess I got what I deserved for driving away my last husband and trying to blame all my problems on everyone. I might as well just kill myself, or just sit home and wait to die. I was worthless in my own eyes.

I couldn't pay my bills, despite the job, and I finally did something I never thought I would have to do; something I had previously thought only ignorant and careless people did – I filed for bankruptcy. That was probably the lowest point of my life. I'd made a lot of mistakes, but the one thing I could pride myself on was that I'd *always* paid my bills. My credit was good, and I'd been taught from an early age just how important that was. I'd pretty much ruined my romantic and social future as I saw it then, and now I was ruining my financial future, too – at least for the next ten years, which is the length of time it would be before it was off my credit report.

The court hearing was humiliating. I felt like I was being judged by people I didn't even know and found to be a bad person because I'd shirked my responsibilities. I was either too lazy to work hard enough to pay my bills, or I was simply incapable of controlling my spending. Neither one of these things was true but I wasn't given the chance to explain, and it probably wouldn't have mattered anyway. I was asked whether I could pay my credit card debt, and I said no. It was thousands of dollars at very high interest rates, and I was making minimum wage. I signed forms saying I would keep paying on my trailer and on my used car, and they stamped the bankruptcy declaration and said they would send me a copy. That was that. Easy to do, but hard to get over.

The only advantage, I suppose, was that I was completely forced to live within my means. I hated it. I was broke, and I was lonely, and I had a dead-end, low-paying job. My parents seemed to have finally gotten tired of helping me along, and they weren't offering me the kind of support they used to. I ate dinner there every night and they watched my daughter while I worked, but I wasn't offered any money, and I wasn't offered any help to get medication or therapy for the panic attacks and depression I still struggled with on a nearly daily basis. They just kept sweeping my problems under the rug, in the 'if you ignore it, it'll go away' style of living. In all fairness, they were probably tired of bailing me out and wanted me to stand on my own. But I wasn't used to it, and I took it as a sign they didn't love me as much as they used to, or they were tired of me and all my screw-ups.

I had to find a way to get out of the financial situation I was in. I was twenty-six years old, and this was not where I'd planned to be in my life, and it was all everybody else's fault...which meant I needed to find someone else to fix it. I wanted to go back to school and finish my degree but I couldn't afford to and my parents weren't offering to pay this time, so I needed someone who would. I thought about it for a few weeks and came to a decision. The next day at work I called Max, after looking up his phone number through information. I told him I was divorced from Alex, and I embellished all the horrible things he had done and how he left me – as if they weren't bad enough on their own. I didn't mention the panic attacks, the dysautonomia, and the crippling depression. I thought he might see them as weaknesses and a turn-off. Before I could chicken out, I boldly just asked if we could pick up where we left off. To my surprise, he said yes. We could. That weekend I drove the twenty miles from my trailer to his house, and started on the next adventure – one that would ultimately culminate in marriage number four.

What I Did Wrong
- Married someone I'd only known for a few months, who I'd started living with almost right away.
- Mingled my finances with those of a man who often spent everything he made.
- Didn't listen to my 'gut instinct' that something wasn't right.
- Wanted my daughter to have a stepfather so badly that I didn't take the time to find the *right* person for that role.
- Potentially put my young child in danger from someone who saw her as an easy target.
- Drove someone out of my life by being horrible, rather than being honest and simply telling him it was over, just so my parents wouldn't be angry with me.
- Avoided going to the doctor for a medical problem because my parents didn't seem 'worried enough' about me and weren't offering to pay for it.
- Ruined my good credit rating because I was selfish, allowed my husband to control me, and didn't want to do the work to pay the debt off once he was gone.
- Was careless enough to drink too much and go home with a man I really knew almost nothing about.
- Went from getting divorced to dating to jumping right into yet another serious relationship because I couldn't stand to be alone.

What To Look For
- Manipulating the people around you so they only see the side of you that you create or want them to see.
- 'Falling in love' right away.
- Deciding you're getting married and going through with it even when you see the problems that are developing.
- Drinking too much or using any kind of drugs that impair your judgment.
- Continuing to see and spend time with people even though they mistreat you, so you don't have to be alone.

- 'Red flags' like your child shying away from a person and not wanting to spend time with him/her, even after knowing that person for a while.
- Lying to yourself about what's taking place in your life so you don't have to work to change anything.
- Ignoring *any* potentially serious medical condition – mental or physical – because no one around you seems to think it's worth worrying over.

What The Therapist Says

We have spent a lot of time exploring the roots for codependent attitudes and relationship addiction. But why is it so hard to break from these attitudes and habits once they are established? Many believe that simply by understanding the reasons for a problem they automatically gain the ability to overcome it. If only it were that simple. Many a person with a serious substance or behavior addiction will be able to attest that "knowing" is only the first step of many in recovery. Being able to not only understand but accept this fact is, in actuality, one of the next important steps to dealing with codependency, and it is not as easy as it may sound.

Let us take a look at why it is so difficult, even after realizing our self-destructive relationship habits, to break the patterns that cause us all this emotional pain. As mentioned earlier codependency and relationship behavior is learned by internalizing what we see our parents and society teaching us about ourselves and the world. The result is not "just" an attitude to be codependent on external validation. This growing up process is what gives us our understanding of who we are and what our place in the universe is; basically our identity.

Again, people may wonder why a person suffering from a low self-image that causes him or her to engage in painful and addictive relationships will not simply change those views that create all this pain. Consider how long and arduous a process it is for us to actually get our sense of self. Growing up and making it through adolescence is a process fraught with emotional pain and struggle at the best of times. The end-product of that lengthy growth process is the sense of identity we carry around within us through most of our lives. It takes a long time and the suffering of lots of emotional turmoil to get to this point. For most, the identity that has been formed at the end of adolescence is something we have fought and worked hard for, however painful the end result may be.

The subconscious mind works in a number of peculiar ways. One of its greatest desires is to minimize pain and maximize happiness. Note that the term "pain" does not distinguish between physical or emotional distress as far as the subconscious is concerned. To it, all pain is pain. Consider again how long and painful the growing up process is that results in our sense of identity, and one can get an idea of how unwilling the subconscious mind might be to have to go through that process all over again. It would rather face the "lesser" pain of being codependent than the prospect of having to relive adolescence. Another important aspect to remember about the subconscious mind is that it has no real imagination, at least not in the sense of "original" thought. All it has is memory. And from that memory the subconscious forms all its expectations of the future, which means that to it all attempts to change our own sense of self are "expected" to be as potentially painful and difficult as the first time we had to go through that process. It cannot imagine that there might be a different way to arrive at a fully formed sense of self.

Keep in mind that most of these avoidance processes never reach our conscious awareness and you will begin to appreciate how difficult it is for an individual suffering from codependence, even if that individual is aware of the predicament, to actually start working on his or her sense of worth. It is just assumed to be easier to look for a better partner or other external source of self-validation. The sad part in this scenario is that the same process that gives us our sense of self also supplies our views of what is "needed" in an external validation source to fill that emotional hole we have inside. These same expectations are often just as flawed as our idea of us being of low intrinsic worth. They set us up for repeated disappointments as the outside sources or partners we engage in to feel "whole" continually fail to supply us with the feeling of worth we need.

One other aspect that serves as a hindrance to us trying to change the way we automatically feel about ourselves also deals with the expectations our subconscious mind holds. It assumes that any process required to change our self-image will take as long as it did to originally form that first but flawed identity. At the same time, our lack of unconditional self-love makes us feel pain right here and now. That immediate pain spurs our subconscious to try to get rid of the pain's source as quickly as possible. When we step on a tack we do not want to wait a week until we can remove it, we want to pull it out *now*. This need to escape our hurt as quickly as possible makes the prospect of a lengthy healing process even less attractive to our subconscious mind. As a result many a person suffering from codependence or relationship addiction will feel a profound lack of patience when it comes to satisfying emotional needs.

Frequently a relationship addict will immediately start daydreaming about a better relationship, either one from past experience or one projected into the future, when the current one does not supply the emotional fuel the addict's self-worth needs. This is also at the root of the addict spending little time after a failed relationship to look for another person. He or she wants to engage in a new relationship as quickly as possible. The emotional pain is immediate and the subconscious wants to feel better right here, right now. This lack of patience makes it difficult for us to want to face those internal attitudes, which cause our emotional yearnings to begin with. We do not want a difficult, lengthy remedy. We want to feel better immediately. But this lack of patience is natural. It is not some sort of profound personality defect. The desire to avoid pain as quickly and efficiently as possible is one of the most basic human traits.

Thankfully, a codependent's chance for recovery is not as dire as our subconscious mind may expect it to be. Just because we have had certain experiences in the past does not make it inevitable that future experiences will turn out the same. While the subconscious mind does not agree with this logical assumption, it is still true. In a manner of speaking, the subconscious is completely impervious to reasonable argument. The only things it believes in are memory and direct experience. Again, do not be discouraged by this fact. The situation is much more hopeful than it may seem. As a matter of fact, the subconscious' limitation to learning from experience only will be one of the major tools we can use to change our unhealthy patterns of thought and behavior. And the beauty of some of these techniques, to be discussed in the following chapters, is that they supply immediate gratification, which is so often a driving force for addictive behaviors.

Most of the methods outlined later will have certain things in common. The first one is that they will aim at changing our expectations for what makes us content. One example in this chapter, in which the author felt discontent, was when the process of getting engaged did not measure up to what she had expected. Note how the failure of reality to live up to what she automatically assumed was to be the "right" way an engagement was to work caused immediate disappointment. But was it the engagement itself that caused that disappointment? Not really. What initiated the feelings of disappointment was the assumption of the subconscious that only a certain pattern of engagement, in this case more pomp and circumstance, would fit the "mold."

In essence, the author's subconscious mind had a concept of what a proper engagement was to be like. This concept was another external factor that could have supplied her with a greater sense of self-worth. If she had a decent engagement then that would be an outside validation of her own worth in the universe. The lack of this "proper" engagement to manifest itself then served as an absence of external validation, or even "proof" for the author's own sense of being someone undesirable or below "average worth." It is very important to realize how external events are used by a codependent person to gauge their assumed personal value. In the chapters to come we will deal with finding immediate sources for self-validation that do not depend on outside events or people. Thus we will begin to overcome our dependency on external factors in order to feel content with who we are.

Chapter 6: Marriage Number Four – Mr. Nice Guy

With Max I did do one thing right – I waited longer to get married. Of course, that was mostly his doing and not mine. We dated for over a year and a half before we stood before family and friends and exchanged those already familiar words. During the time we dated we never fought. Not once. We had little disagreements, but they were nothing serious. Once he got upset because I talked too much about a male co-worker, and I'm sure I got aggravated by him once or twice, but I really thought we could be happy together. After all, he was always happy, or at least it seemed that way on the outside. We went places together, went out to dinner, went shopping on the weekends, and did all kinds of things that young couples do. And I respected him. He didn't kiss on the first date, he didn't sleep around, and he knew what he wanted from a relationship. I couldn't help but admire that. He had a nice house in a good part of town and he had a steady, intellectual, well-paying job. He'd never been married, and he liked kids – including Karyn, who was already growing up so quickly it seemed like every time I blinked she'd changed.

After dating for about a year I was starting to get restless. It was the same old thing. We didn't live together, he refused to stay the night at my trailer – although I could stay at his house if I liked and I could even bring Karyn. It made me feel like my trailer just wasn't good enough for him. There was no ring on my hand and no talk of marriage. I hadn't met his parents or siblings or friends. I'd managed to keep the 'what ifs' at bay for a while, but they were starting up again. What if I wasn't good enough? What if he was seeing someone else? What if he dumped me? What if he decided he didn't want the 'package deal' after all? What if he was ashamed of me? I don't know why I thought those things. He was always kind and thoughtful to everyone, and I'd felt safe and comfortable with him for months. He even regularly gave me money so I could afford to go back to school. He paid my tuition and handed me some extra cash to help cover my bills. I excelled in school. My panic attacks had gone into remission and I no longer felt depressed. I played with my daughter again. I was happy…except I wasn't. Not really. Not deep down inside where it counted. If he loved me he should want to marry me, and he didn't. I agonized over how to get what I needed from him or from someone else, if it came to that. Whatever it took to get that critical validation I was missing.

Frustrated, I accepted a girls-night-out invitation with an old friend from high school who I'd vaguely kept in touch with. Max didn't seem to mind. Occasionally we did our own thing on the weekends and didn't see one another. At a karaoke bar late that night I kept feeling like I was being watched. I searched the crowd through the smoke and haze, and I finally realized it was Lee, watching me from another table where he sat with a pissed-off-looking blonde. Oops. Was he really watching me? Was that what had made her so angry? I felt a haughty sense of satisfaction at that. He came to the table and we made small talk for a few minutes, and then he went back to his date. Shortly afterward, they left together. I sighed. So much for thinking I was better than that heavily made up, over-fluffed, over-dyed, over-bosomed bimbo I'd seen him with. I'd really missed him, and I didn't realize how much until I saw him again, with someone else. Maybe he was just what I needed. When I was seeing Lee before, I hadn't been willing to see Max as well. It didn't seem fair to them, and it was too complicated for me. Based on the prudish way I was raised, it smacked of sluttiness. Now, I thought it might be OK after all. My opinions on life were slowly changing, and they no longer completely mirrored my parents' beliefs, although they were still surprisingly close. Lee was easygoing, Max was easygoing. As long as I wasn't sleeping with both of them I wasn't a whore, right?

My friend and I left shortly after that and Lee was in the parking lot, without his date, waiting for me. Looks like I had 'won' after all. I was headed to my friend's house...could he come, too? It was only a few blocks, and we all congregated in her kitchen. I was leaning against the wall, watching Lee set a six-pack on the counter. He walked over, looked me up and down, said "God, I missed you," and kissed me thoroughly before I had a chance to say anything. He couldn't stay long, and I fell asleep on the couch from all the beer I'd drunk at the bar. He left his phone number, and I called him the next day and went to his house for a while. He wanted to keep seeing me, and I eagerly agreed. That night I was going to Max's house for dinner, and I was going to tell him I thought we should back off a bit, and start seeing other people. I still wanted to see him, just not exclusively. I still wanted his money, you see. I wanted the safety and security, and to be able to go out and have more fun as well. I wanted someone to pay my way so I could go off and do something else. I was excited about spending time with Lee. It was familiar and comfortable, like going home again...but of course you can't really do that, can you?

When I got to Max's house, he was sitting on his roof. He said it was his thinking spot, but I'd never seen him up there before. My brain told me to get ready. I was suddenly seized with the certainty that he was going to break up with me, saying our relationship had gotten stale and it was time to go our separate ways. I didn't want him to do that. I wanted both Max and Lee. Lee provided me with fun and easygoing enjoyment. Max provided me with stability, and money, and nice dinners, and the kinds of things I couldn't get on my own, and he treated Karyn well, playing with her for hours. It wasn't just his money I was attracted to, but that was certainly part of it. No point in lying about it. It was nice not to have to struggle. I still didn't have much, but I was able to quit working and go to school full-time on Max's money and a grant I'd obtained, which meant I could get done faster and wouldn't have to pay anything back. I finished up the few classes I needed for my two-year degree, and then I went on to a four-year degree. My degree would be in Legal Administration, and I envisioned getting a great, high-paying corporate law firm job with my bachelor's degree. I really didn't have a clue how virtually worthless two-year and even many four-year degrees were becoming in many types of jobs. Just about everybody had one. Had I known that, it might have dampened my spirits and I might have forgotten all about finishing my schooling, but I was blissfully unaware.

Max came down from the roof and we walked down his road, glancing warily at each other.

"I want to talk to you about something," he finally said.

I told him I wanted to talk to him, too, but he should go first. I guessed that if he dumped me, at least I wouldn't have to worry about telling him about Lee. He nodded, and we walked in silence for a couple of minutes, my heart pounding. I felt miserable. The panic attacks that had left me alone for the last few months were threatening to come back, and I could feel one lurking there, just on the edge, waiting for a chance to terrify me again. I just knew Max was through with me. Of course I wasn't good enough for him! How could I have ever thought I was? I wondered what had made him decide. Was it something specific I had done? Some stupid thing I had said? Something else I had failed at? My thoughts were moving so fast I almost didn't catch it when he took a deep breath and said "What would you think about getting engaged?" Huh? Had I heard him right? Here I was so sure I was unworthy of his affection, and I'd come down here to say I thought we should cool things for a while, and now he was dangling a marriage proposal in my face.

The smart thing to do would be to say no, and to be honest, and to say that I needed more time, so of course I didn't do that. I told him I thought it was a wonderful idea. I threw my arms around him and almost knocked him over in my enthusiasm. I laughed until I cried. All I could think about were wedding bells. The ring, the dress, the church, the invitations! It was all so exciting! I'd make it work this time. I'd show everybody I could do it, and my dad would be proud of me and I'd feel like I mattered. The next day I sent Lee an email and told him about the proposal. I haven't heard from him since. The following weekend, Max and I had an out-of-town trip scheduled, and while we were there we went ring shopping.

The ring was too big since my hands are very small, and it had to be reduced in size. When it came back from the jeweler, Max wouldn't let me wear it. He just shook his head and smiled. The next time he came to my house he brought the ring, and he gave it to me, and he got down on one knee and recited a poem that he had *written and memorized* just for me. The idea that he'd taken the time to do that meant the world to me. *That* was what I was looking for, and I became even more certain I was doing the right thing this time. He was perfect. Of course he wasn't really perfect, but I was having a difficult time finding anything wrong with him at that moment. I couldn't see anything but how happy we would be.

Planning the wedding went smoothly. I moved into his home, and my parents sold their trailer and mine, which were located about thirty minutes away, and moved into a new home just over a mile from Max's. They didn't even want to be half an hour from me, and from their granddaughter. They had to be closer. Whether it was out of loneliness, curiosity, or control, I don't know. Probably a little bit of all of them – and I know there was a lot of love mixed in there, as well. They were used to running my life, at least in the sense that I was so concerned with what they thought I always tried to please them and I agonized over doing things I knew or thought they wouldn't like.

Looking back on it I'm not so sure they ever *really* tried to run my life. I think I just took their opinions as gospel, did what they suggested out of a fear of upsetting them, and then blamed them for not 'letting me' do it my way. What I wanted was for them to agree with everything I said and read my mind, so they gave me the answers I wanted to hear as 'their opinion.' Just one more way I tried to sabotage my relationships. Max and I had started going to church together, and we had our ceremony there. It was the first time I'd ever been married in a 'real' church. I figured a soldier's chapel, a Vegas wedding chapel, and an outdoor amphitheater didn't really count, and I saw my marriage to Max as my first 'real' marriage. The others were simply practice runs. Dress rehearsals, if you will. Anything I could do to justify it. Anything I could think of in order to make myself feel less guilty, or distract myself from the fact that I was doing this – *again* – with more fear and trepidation than I felt I should have on what was supposed to be a happy day.

In all honesty, I felt better about that marriage than I had about any of the previous ones, but I still didn't feel right. It seemed too much like I was doing it because he'd asked and I couldn't bear to say no. Was I being fair to him? I just didn't know. He really was a sweet guy, and he deserved a woman who was truly in love with him. I did *love* him, but I wasn't *in love* with him...and I wasn't willing to break his heart by refusing his proposal. So we went through with the wedding and we moved on to the business of building a life together. Perhaps I would fall 'in love' in the process. I didn't. Not really. But we had a lot of fun for about the first year or so. It was clear we genuinely cared for one another. I stayed in school, intent on getting my bachelors degree, and I took a job writing for an Internet company. I'd written a few articles for local newspapers in the past and had enjoyed it, so I started doing some of that again. It helped me make a little bit of income, and Max's job supplied everything we needed. We weren't rich by any means but I wasn't poor any more, either, and that was a great weight off my shoulders. I was able to start rebuilding my credit through the use of his credit cards, and that gave me a better feeling of security.

After about a year we started to fight more. Little things began to get to us, and we got aggravated with each other pretty easily. I thought he was too prudish about how he wanted his life to go, and he wasn't willing to take enough risks. He didn't seem to like change very much, and I didn't want to have to conform to his schedule. He had his opinions, too. I didn't make enough extra money for the amount I was spending, I slept too late on the weekends, I didn't know how to cook, I wasn't much of a housekeeper, I wasn't affectionate enough. The list was long. To be fair, I *was* spending a lot of money. I suppose the rest was a matter of perspective. He was used to being a bachelor, and he'd lived on his own for some time. He was set in his ways. He had a routine, and getting married – especially to someone with a young child – had disrupted that. I think he enjoyed it for a while but it was getting old for him, and it was getting old for me, too. I felt trapped yet again. I wasn't looking for another man or anything, I just wanted to be on my own. With all the marriages and other relationships, and with my parents being so close to me, I'd never really had the opportunity to live on my own, to actually have a home on my own terms. I wondered what kind of example I was setting for my daughter.

She had trouble in school with socialization, she cried easily, and she didn't talk much, to me or anyone else. Was that just her nature, or had I caused that? I didn't know, and I wasn't sure how to find out – or even if I *could* find out. She said she was happy, but I could see she wasn't. Anyone could've seen that. She was withdrawn most of the time, and I was pretty sure she was being teased at school, just like I had been when I was young. Because she wouldn't talk to me about it I couldn't make much headway. I received at least one phone call every school year from an allegedly 'concerned' teacher who was asking a lot of nosy questions. The school psychologist even called me and wanted to know what my daughter's home life was like. I told her in a kind of careful way that it wasn't any of her damn business. I was offended, and I was annoyed that someone who knew nothing about me or my daughter or our lives outside of her school day would presume to judge that something was wrong with the way I was raising her. How *dare* they question what kind of mother I was! I took it personally, and I felt I was being accused of something I hadn't done. She didn't have a bad home life at all. It did go through my head that she might have been a little traumatized over the multiple marriages. But she had been so young…did she even really remember living with her father or her first stepfather? I wasn't willing to really entertain the thought that anything I had done could have caused her to be this way.

She still saw her father only rarely, and she never saw Alex. She didn't even know about my first marriage, back when I was seventeen. So how much was my fault and how much was just her personality? I couldn't answer that, and since I couldn't answer it I shoved it out of my mind. I tried to get closer to her and be more of a mother to her…and more of a friend. She resisted. She acted like the stereotypical teenager, but she was only nine. Add to that the fact she was very intellectual and wise beyond her years, and she had started to develop so early that older boys were noticing her and kids her age were pointing at her expanding chest and giggling. By the time she was in third grade I was buying her baggy shirts to hide it, and her bra size was larger than anyone in our immediate family. She was embarrassed and uncomfortable in her own skin, and she didn't know how to cope with it. I wondered sometimes what I was going to do about her, but I kept trying to forget about it and do something else. I wanted to help her, but only if it didn't take up too much of my time and effort. I loved her, but I was still a selfish person at heart. I didn't understand why the world wasn't simply handing me everything I wanted and taking care of my problems for me. I thought I deserved at least that much for all the suffering I'd been through at the hands of others.

On top of my concerns about Karyn, I wanted to put in a pool and take a trip and do some other fun things, and

Maximillian refused. We didn't have the money, he said. The bank balance and our credit availability said otherwise, but since he was the one making the largest share of the income by far, there wasn't much I could do about it. It upset me, and I made it known, which led to more fights between us. I shouldn't have been complaining. All my needs were met, and most of my wants were met. He even bought me a brand new car he said was just for me, and then after the deal was done he forbade me to smoke in it. It was my contingency car – contingent upon a lack of nicotine whilst behind the wheel. I almost told him to take it back, but the allure of the leather seats and big engine and new car smell was too much to walk away from, and I caved in. I already didn't smoke in our home, and now I couldn't smoke in my car. Eventually I quit altogether, only to go back to it a few months later when the fighting got worse and the depression started to creep back in.

In the evenings, when we really should have been spending time as a family, Max usually played video games, read, or watched TV in the living room, Karyn watched TV in her room, and I sat on the front porch with my cigarettes and a book, swatting at mosquitoes. Not exactly one big happy family. My mom usually came over every evening for an hour or so, and I stopped by my parents' house and saw my dad once or twice a week, sometimes more. Just like with Alex, Max and I were together in the same house but we weren't really together as a cohesive unit. We didn't fight as much as Alex and I had, but we mostly just didn't say anything at all to each other, other than the day Max told me if he knew what I was really like, he would never have married me. Ouch. That was painful, and just when I was starting to feel safe; resigned to a slightly boring and routine existence, but still safe. It was clear that he felt he'd made a mistake, but he didn't seem interested in getting a divorce. We actually talked about it, and the consensus was he didn't like giving up his space and routine, and I'd never been able to have my own space. We both had our problems with the living arrangement we'd gotten ourselves into, but we also both cared very much for each other, and we weren't sure what to do about it.

After much discussion, it was decided we would live apart but stay married. Max said he would pay off my car so I wouldn't have a payment on it, and he would pay all my bills except my house payment, which I would be responsible for. That was a *more* than generous offer. How could I refuse? We would continue to have our joint tax returns and our healthcare, so that was no longer an issue for me and I wouldn't have to go back onto the welfare system for medical coverage. It was a tremendously good deal, and one most people in my situation would never get. I was able to have my cake and eat it, too, and I set about checking with lenders regarding housing and looking to see what kinds of options were out there. Through doing all that, I found there was just one problem…in order for me to get a house of my own, I had to have Max sign the loan papers as well, since we were married. He balked at that. What if I just stopped paying? He would be responsible for two homes and it could damage his credit, not to mention cut into his savings and investments. He refused to do it at all. He wouldn't even consider it.

I told him the only other way for us to live apart was to get a divorce. He shrugged. Whatever I wanted to do was fine with him. We could get divorced and just date each other again, but if we divorced he wasn't paying my bills. I negotiated for at least the payoff on the car, over $20,000, which I got. It was mine, free and clear. I promptly turned around and sold it to buy something a lot cheaper, and put the extra money in the bank. I filed for divorce. Max was not happy, and looking back on it I can't blame him. It was kind of a lousy thing to do. I had gone into 'look out for myself' mode, and that was all I was thinking about. I guess that wasn't a good choice, and it must have been a lot more stress than I realized, because my panic attacks came back in full force. I started shaking again, and my heart would skip and race, skip and race. I had no money to go to the doctor, so I tried to just live my life the best I could. I had trouble eating, and I lost weight again. I worried about the health effects of that, and the worry that I might really be damaging my health and my body only succeeded in making the panic attacks and depressive episodes worse.

Karyn and I shared a bedroom at Max's house, my parents gave me the deed to the half-acre of land next door to them for a dollar, and I had a house built on it, back when real estate prices were really, really low. I definitely lucked into the loan, since I had a recent bankruptcy on my credit, was newly divorced, and was self-employed and not yet well-established in my full-time writing career – all strikes against me when it came to qualifying for a loan. I didn't think I'd be able to get it at all without my dad co-signing, but I did. It was the first thing (other than a credit card) that I ever qualified for on my own, and I was proud of that accomplishment if nothing else.

Just for the record, I really didn't want to live next to my parents again. I loved them, and I still do, but they had such a hold over my life…and as I've alluded to before, I don't know that they necessarily meant to. I think it was more just a routine we'd fallen into throughout the years, left over from my childhood. I didn't know how to break it, and I didn't think I could afford to buy a house somewhere else. Them giving me that land not only secured me a down payment with the lender, but it also made how much I had to borrow significantly less than it would have otherwise been. Without that, I would've been stuck renting somewhere, or buying a super-cheap house in a really lousy neighborhood. I was promised privacy when I agreed to take the lot and build there, but of course I didn't get it. My dad was there all the time while the house was being built, just watching to make sure the workers didn't screw something up. Once the house was done my mom wandered over several times a day, just to see what I was doing. It wasn't really a problem, and yet it was. I couldn't decide. I was grateful for it and aggravated by it at the same time; torn between thinking they were looking out for me because they cared and thinking they were always watching me because they didn't believe I could be trusted to survive on my own. Did I mention I was becoming a little paranoid?

I had my own space, but I still couldn't be my own person. If I left in my car, mom would call my cell phone to see where I was going. If I wanted to have someone over, I couldn't do it without my parents' knowledge. I still ate dinner with my parents every night. The only reason I had a kitchen at all was because it had come with the house. Other than using the refrigerator and the microwave, I didn't need it for anything. But it was still mine. All mine. Karyn and I moved into our new home just a week before she turned ten years old. So much space! And we could do whatever we wanted to do with it. Naturally, we proceeded to fill it full of things we didn't need and couldn't really afford, leaving me with another round of credit card debt on top of my house payment. Max came over each weekend, and we went and did things together. We were divorced and dating one another, which was strange, but also fun. It was the only time Karyn and I really did anything together. Max helped me set up my house because my anxiety and depression were getting so bad it was hard for me to do much. Thank God I could work from home! That was the only thing that saved me financially. There was no way I would've been able to hold down what I called a 'real job' – the traditional, out-of-the-house, work-with-customers kind of thing.

I still got calls from the school about my daughter's withdrawn behavior, and I still panicked almost every day...sometimes several times in one day. I had very little energy, and I had to force myself to do enough writing to pay the bills. I was vaguely worried about everything, and I had trouble putting my finger on just what the problem was. I guess it boiled down to the fact that I wasn't really *living* – I was mostly just *existing.* Anyone who has done both will tell you they are far from the same thing. Going out with Max started to get on my nerves. I don't even know why. Maybe the idea of dating my ex-husband just got too bizarre, or maybe we were just growing apart even more than we had while we were married. I'm not sure. All I know is I was again looking for a change.

Somewhere along the way our dating relationship morphed into a good friendship. It was better that way. We could still hang out and do things, but there was no pressure for anything else. He finally started dating other people, and we stopped spending as much time together. I didn't have much interest in the dating scene. Oh, I went out a couple of times, but it wasn't a big deal. They were men I met on the Internet through a dating site, and I was thoroughly unimpressed by any of them. It's amazing how people lie on the Internet! Guys who said they were 'average build' were fifty pounds overweight, guys who said they had good jobs were 'between opportunities,' people were late showing up, they wanted me to pay their way, they had five kids and wanted more, they weren't *actually* divorced yet, they had some bizarre fetish, they only liked to talk about themselves, and the list went on and on. It was terrible. I became convinced this was my penance for my multiple marriages, and I became very worried about panicking when I was out with someone new. How would I explain that?

My overactive imagination could see it all…I would be stuck in my home, riddled with bedsores from never moving off the couch, panicking every day over pointless thoughts and feelings, and sinking deeper into depression, all alone when my daughter grew up and moved on – and who could blame her for wanting to get the hell out? I hadn't been much of a mother. I would grow old and feeble, after taking care of my parents twenty-four hours a day in their old age. I would die and no one would notice or care and my pets would eat me for sustenance. Maybe someone from the bank would find my mummified and dog-chewed remains when I stopped paying my bills. Maybe I'd be one of those old ladies who broke out in chronic cats, letting them cover every available surface until my house became one giant litter box. I didn't have a very high opinion of myself or of my future. When I sat and took stock of my life, I didn't see much of a point to it.

Sure I had a decent house in an OK neighborhood, but I was struggling to pay for it. My car was older even though it ran well. I had no real money, and no real prospects of any. My writing had stagnated – I didn't want to spend the rest of my life writing only what others wanted me to write. I wanted to create something of my own.

At night I had trouble sleeping. When I did sleep I dreamed of horrible things. Nightmares where I died and no one cared. Nightmares where I killed my daughter, or someone else did. Nightmares where I just lived on and on and on in a kind of miserable existence and couldn't seem to just die properly. It was horrible and I dreaded sleeping because of it, but I was so very tired all the time. I saw it in my daughter, too. She was lethargic, and her schoolwork was not as good as it used to be. She started staying up very late, unable to sleep, and she ate more and more, getting chubby and unhealthy. She complained every time she had to go to see her father, but she complained when he didn't call for a long time. Didn't he care about her?

The teachers called me more often – she was crying in class, she refused to do her work, she wouldn't answer questions, she didn't have any friends, she looked different from the others, she acted oddly. I didn't know what to tell them. How could I explain about all the failed marriages and the sadness and the upset; the turmoil that my life – and by extension hers – had become? I didn't have the strength to deal with it, so I told them she seemed just fine at home, and I knew some kids were teasing her, and that was probably what was bothering her most of the time. I said her father ignored her and wasn't in her life. I blamed it on everything and everyone I could and made it sound like I was a sainted mother, doing everything I possibly could do in a world that was working against me. I couldn't possibly let others think I was doing anything wrong. I wasn't raised to admit to making mistakes. Come to think of it, I didn't even *make* mistakes. I was better than that. I knew that was a lie, but I refused to openly acknowledge it. If I ignored it, it would eventually go away.

She didn't seem 'fine' at home, but I didn't know how to deal with that, either. My own mother and father had mostly swept my problems under the rug, so I did the same thing with Karyn's difficulties. I was preprogrammed to do it that way. We talked only about trivial things, and we left the rest alone. She spent most of her time in her room with the door closed, and I spent most of my time on my couch, half-ass working while I watched whatever garbage was on television. Eventually, my parents started to nag me. Karyn seemed depressed…she was getting heavy, and she really had a bad attitude. She should find an activity or a hobby – something she enjoyed doing. I knew deep down they were right, but to be honest I didn't care that much. One evening I said something off-handed to Karyn about it. She seemed to perk up a bit.

"Could I take martial arts?" she asked me.

I was surprised, since she'd never shown much interest in doing anything like that before. I thought about it for a few minutes and decided it would be fine, with the exception of paying for it. I would have to know how much it would cost, and whether we could afford it. Otherwise, I thought it would be a great idea. It would teach her a valuable safety skill, and it was great exercise. I had taken some martial arts training when I was younger, and I really liked it. I only stopped because we moved away. That weekend we did some checking around, and we couldn't find much we liked. The next weekend, we went again. Finally, we stopped at a place in a neighboring town, about twenty minutes from the house. Max had come with us that day, and he was interested in joining up, too. The guy running the dojo gave us a great deal. Even though we weren't technically still a family he would give us a family discount, making it much cheaper. We signed up, got Max and Karyn both uniforms and white belts, and got ready to go to class the following Monday. We went home and she told my parents about it, and they offered to pay half the fee, with Max paying the other half. I was free and clear, other than the gasoline I would use to drive her back and forth four nights a week.

The class really seemed to help her feel better. She was stiff and sore the first week or two, but after that it was easier for her to do the exercises that were required. She didn't exactly make friends, but I did catch her occasionally speaking to someone else or at least smiling or nodding an acknowledgment to them. And of course she talked to Max all the time. I think she felt safe there when he was in class. She genuinely liked him, and she was old enough to actually get to know him and understand what kind of person he was, instead of seeing him as her ex-stepfather. Instead, he was just her friend. I was happy with the arrangement, and each night while she was in class my mother (who almost always came with us) and I would walk down the plaza near the dojo and go into stores, looking at clothes, books, household goods, and tiny puppies and kittens in the pet shop. It gave us both something to do, and it forced me to get out of my own head a little bit.

I was still panicky sometimes, but not as badly, and both Karyn and I seemed to be a little less depressed. Life was not perfect by any stretch of the imagination, but we laughed more and we talked to one another more. At home she practiced her martial arts moves on me and showed off for her grandpa. He enjoyed it, and it made her smile. Life was starting to return to some semblance of 'good,' but something was missing. I was starting to realize how alone I was, and how lonely I was getting at night, by myself in that big bed with no one around. I needed something new in my life. Instead of hunting for a man, I traded cars. I sold my old Monte Carlo to a young guy on the next block, and I bought an old Porsche. I'd wanted one since high school, in the late eighties. The only one I could afford had been driven hard since the late eighties, and had some serious issues. I got it cheap and thought I could fix it up. I couldn't. Neither could anyone else I knew without some serious money – much more than the car was worth.

I got rid of it by trading it on an old Corvette. I'd always wanted one. When I was younger I'd told myself my definition of 'making it' was a Corvette and a Rolex watch. I managed to get both – a used Corvette from a small car dealer in a neighboring town, and a used Rolex watch from a seller on an online auction site. I drove the Corvette for about three months, until the clutch went out and I had to have it replaced. It wasn't cheap, and the mechanic said it also wasn't the first clutch replacement that car had been through. How nice. I wish the dealer had told me that, but he probably didn't know either. After I got the new clutch I realized I wasn't really that happy with the car. Who knew what would break next? It was uncomfortable to get in and out of, and I couldn't carry hardly anything in it. Plus, I kept scraping it on the ground trying to get around driveways and parking lots. In the end, the Corvette was just a car and the Rolex was just a watch. No one but me really gave a damn about my timepiece or my vehicle. I sold them both and financed a brand new, mid-priced convertible. Add that car payment to the house payment and credit card bills. Oh, and I had finally finished my schooling, attaining a four-year degree in Legal Administration, so I had student loans to repay as well. Max had stopped paying for school when we divorced. I'd started making tolerable money but things were still stretched tight, and since I was self-employed I was always working. Free time where I didn't have *anything* to do was almost non-existent.

I seemed to *find* the free time, though, to get myself involved with a married man who came to the dojo. It wasn't some kind of torrid affair. It was mostly just two lonely people spending a little more time together than they needed to, and getting a little closer to one another than they really ought to…and when he started pushing for too much physically I broke it off. I thought I was learning. 'See?' I told myself. 'I didn't sleep with him, and I broke it off when it became clear that was all he wanted, and that having him divorce his wife was not an option.' I didn't want to play the other woman again. I had done that enough in the past, and it gets old very quickly. I was proud of myself for finally – I thought – realizing just having a man, any man, wasn't enough. And then I made my biggest mistake – one that could have cost me my life.

What I Did Wrong
- Married someone primarily for the money and stability he offered.
- Accepted a marriage proposal because it was there, when I'd originally planned to back away from the exclusivity of the relationship and see other people.
- Ignored what was wrong with my daughter because I didn't want to deal with it or admit that I might have caused it – following my parents' attitude of sweeping problems under the rug.
- Lied to the school about what was taking place at home, just to make sure I made myself look good.
- Swindled my soon-to-be-ex out of the money he used to pay off the car, by paying the loan off and then selling the car so I got (and kept) most of the money.
- Moved in next door to my parents even though I wanted to be free – it was cheaper, and I didn't want to hurt their feelings.
- Got involved (even though it was brief) with a married man who was very clearly off limits.

What To Look For
- Marrying for anything other than real love (money, safety, security, stability, comfort, etc.).
- Getting married because it has been offered to you, when you weren't sure that was really what you wanted.
- Ignoring the needs of others (especially your children) because you don't want to face your own fears or problems.
- Cheating (emotionally, physically, or financially).
- Letting others control what you're doing, instead of being in charge of your own life.
- Getting involved with people who are bad for you (like people who are already married to someone else, people who do drugs or are alcoholics, abusive people, etc.).
- Living the kind of life that causes intense stress, or that manifests itself in problems like anxiety, panic attacks, and depression.
- Lying to others so that you don't look bad or so you don't have to admit faults or mistakes – or lying to yourself for the same reasons.

What The Therapist Says
This chapter is interesting because it emphasizes a dilemma many relationship addicts experience at some point in their lives. At one point or another, the addict realizes his or her behavior is not healthy, that it's potentially dangerous even, but is at a loss as to what to do differently. They see the way their lives appear to repeat themselves, but since they have never seen or learned any different options of behaving they now feel as if they are stuck doing what they did in the past, even though they know it will not work. This adds another level of frustration, even resignation, to an already emotionally strained situation.

Yet at this stage a codependent will often try to look for anything that could make the new relationship different from the previous one. Differences in the partners or the relationship dynamics are desperately hoped for as a means of breaking the old circle of failed relationships. This shows the drive and desire to improve one's situation. It also underlines the previously stated fact that the subconscious mind is only able to call upon those expectations and behavior alternatives it has learned in the past. The subconscious is unable to creatively come up with and believe in a truly alternative and new way of behaving.

But that does not mean that we cannot find a way to teach this part of our minds new behaviors and alternatives. It is not a question of whether that is possible, but of how to accomplish it. If it were impossible to ever unlearn old patterns of behavior then there would be no hope for anyone to ever make it through an addiction concern of any kind. The mere fact that there are many people who have managed to do just that proves that there are methods of retraining our subconscious to let go of attitudes which repeatedly cause us pain and do not supply us with the happiness we crave from our lives. Again, the issue facing the codependent is not one of whether the process is feasible, but what methods are going to work.

There are actually a number of techniques, a lot of them truly easy, which have been proven helpful in dealing with codependence. Some of them appear so ludicrously simple that many a sufferer from self-worth deficiencies cannot believe they would actually work. Since belief in success makes a big difference in how motivated a codependent relationship addict will be to try these methods of recovery, I want to spend a little time on explaining the theoretical and therapeutic reasoning behind them. Once an individual gets a feeling that means of recovery have scientific grounding he or she is much more willing to utilize them. In a strange way, this very attitude is also a deeply ingrained pattern of subconscious belief that our society tends to impart on us.

First of all I need to reiterate the concept of how our subconscious mind, our attitudes, habits, and our identity are formed and work. As we grow up our subconscious stores memories. Its main function is to act as a vast repertoire of past experiences we can draw upon in order to survive life. But it is more than just a storage bin for memory. As we learn and accumulate memories our subconscious looks for patterns in them. If certain situations repeatedly lead to painful outcomes our subconscious mind will reason that these situations will have to be avoided. Inversely, any behaviors or situations that are connected with a lessening of pain and increases in happiness will cause the subconscious to motivate us to repeat these particular patterns. Those are the two premises on which our automatic attitudes and beliefs are built: the desires to minimize pain and maximize contentment. The result is a deeply ingrained belief about how the world works, what is important, and, most importantly, about how we see our own worth and what makes us happy.

Following this reasoning it is easy to understand how past experiences can shape the way we see life and ourselves. If we continuously experienced rejection from others if we did not conform to them in a certain way our subconscious mind would use that information to shape our innermost attitudes. It may determine that our true views and likes are unwanted by the world and cause us pain if expressed. Therefore, our innermost self must be unwanted and "bad." We then may very well internalize the belief that in order to be happy we have to act in ways that make others like us and must not allow our true feelings and "self" to be recognized. This, in turn, maintains the concept that our innermost self is unlikable, unlovable, and as such of no true "worth."

This is one possible way of how a belief of low self-esteem may be fostered. Other means include upbringings in which the child never has any control over his or her environment, especially in trying to avoid pain and increase happiness. That may lead to an ingrained belief in the child that he is innately helpless and weak, requiring outside sources to secure his happiness and safety. That, again, can then result in a very poor sense of self-worth as weakness usually has a negative and undesirable connotation in our society.

But repeated experiences are not always required to establish a deeply held subconscious belief. If a situation has enough inherent pleasure or pain even a single event can lead our subconscious mind to create an automatic habit of thought and behavior. Severe trauma of any kind is a good example of that. Experiences of rape, tragedy, violence, or severe terror can be so immensely painful that no repetition is required for our innermost beliefs to draw a certain set of conclusions. The feeling of shame and utter worthlessness experienced by rape victims is a good example. Another is the repeated occurrence of post-traumatic stress disorder in war veterans or victims of singularly horrible traumatic events. In these cases it is not repetition but the severity of the pain experienced that leads the subconscious mind to draw its conclusions.

The important part to remember is that the subconscious mind creates these beliefs on the basis of association rather than logical reasoning. If one thing occurs simultaneously with another often enough, it must be connected. This fact makes it very difficult for anyone to try to overcome subconscious beliefs by using reason or internal logical debate. The behaviors are so immediate and automatic we tend to become aware of them only after we have already engaged in them. Or, if we do realize we are about to engage in an old behavior pattern we know does not work, our own internal reasoning is often incapable of stopping us from completing it. That, in turn, will add to any feelings of helplessness and worthlessness we already harbor inside.

Yet in the techniques I will mention in the following chapters we will use the very means by which our subconscious learns, mainly repeated experience, to try to undo those beliefs inside of us that cause us pain and repeated disappointment. On the surface some of these methods may appear childish or improbable. Trust me, they have been proven effective in many a case of codependency or any other situation linked to low internal self-worth. The key to their success is not necessarily belief in them, but repeated application. In a way we will be trying to create new habits within ourselves, and those require repeated use.

Just as we most often do not have to consciously remember all the steps we engage in when brushing and flossing our teeth we will attempt to replace old automatic patterns of thought and action with new ones. Remember how you had to actively remind yourself of what to do the first months of learning to brush your teeth? I would bet that nowadays you do not have to recall the various steps you use in oral hygiene when you step into the bathroom each morning. Those steps have become a subconscious habit. And that is what we will begin to build: new subconscious habits and beliefs that will counteract those behaviors that cause us pain.

Chapter 7: Marriage Number Five - What Was I Thinking?

It was, by far, the shortest marriage in my history – even beating the nine-month time frame of the first one. If you'd been walking by and had accidentally blinked, you'd have missed it. A grand total of five months from the time we said 'I do' until the ink was dry on the divorce papers. It was also the most volatile marriage I had gotten myself into, and I didn't really think about the danger I was in until it was already over with. It was serious denial on a grand scale. Once the dust had settled it was only then that I became really frightened, looking back on the different ways I could have lost my life and the emotional and physical toll those few short months took on Karyn and me. You don't see it when you're in it. You don't realize how bad it really is. Instead, you think it must be normal if *you're* doing it, and there are a lot of other people who are just like you. Part of that is true...there *are* a lot of other people going through marital hell...but that doesn't make it 'normal.'

I'd managed to stay away from any serious relationships for a couple of years, mostly by just keeping to myself, and partially because no new prospects presented themselves. I basically became a recluse, at first because I was still depressed and panicky and then later because I had little money to do anything. I was proud of my ability to be on my own but still ashamed of my past, and I was terribly lonely. I didn't like to talk about my past. Any time I had to disclose it (which thankfully was not often) I always made it sound like it was 'all their fault.' Not to say they never did anything wrong, but I still hadn't come to terms with my own bad choices. I wasn't willing to admit I might have been at least partially at fault with the things I did, or that I might have driven them to do or say some of the things they did or said. I wouldn't even acknowledge that I might have picked men who were not the right choices *for me* – men who were basically just totally incompatible with what I was actually looking for and what I really needed. After I walked away from that married man and felt so proud of my ability to reason that he was a bad choice, it wasn't really that long before I met a single man who wasn't well-liked by the others in the martial arts class. Since I was cultivating such a high opinion of my ability to 'just say no,' I felt safe in getting involved in another relationship. I thought I could handle it now.

I should have known, when everyone else tried to avoid him, that I should have done the same. I should have run, not walked, in the opposite direction. Instead, he intrigued me. Why did people dislike him? He was attractive, with that unique combination of light hair and dark eyes, and he seemed to be very friendly. He had a ready laugh, and he was always trying to talk to people and joke with them and be friends with them. At least that's what I saw at the time. I wonder, if I looked at that same scene through the lens of hindsight, what I would see. Would I see a friendly person, or would I see a desperate person trying way too hard to get people to like him and failing miserably at it? Would I see the same desperate person if I looked at myself through that same lens? I'm not sure I want to know. I already cringe at the memory of some of the things I said and did back then, and I already feel bad enough about it. Seeing what I managed to overlook would likely just make me feel worse. It's over and done with now, and looking back over my shoulder wouldn't solve anything. But I take the memory of how it turned out with me, always, to help protect me from doing it again.

His name was Jack. He was an outcast and an all-around jerk. He was loud, he was obnoxious, and he was a lot like Alex. Of course, I didn't see that then. I thought I had grown and changed so much because I had walked away from Mr. Married a few months before. I was still patting myself on the back, and I thought I knew what I was doing. I didn't see what was wrong with Jack – not because it wasn't there, but because I simply didn't want to see it. Instead, I viewed him as misunderstood and troubled (much like I was, even though I refused to acknowledge it). I wanted to 'save' him – from what, I'm still not sure. From himself, I guess. He didn't take much interest in me and I should have left well-enough alone, but if you've read to this point in the book you already know I couldn't do that. It wasn't something I was very good at. The fact that he ignored me wasn't really that much of a deterrent. Instead, it gave me something I was looking for – a challenge.

I was the one who asked him out. He seemed surprised, but he accepted. We hadn't really talked that much, there hadn't been any flirting going on, and he didn't even know my name! When I came bouncing up to him asking to go for a ride on his motorcycle it took him a minute to figure out just what the hell was going on. You could almost see the gears clashing in his head. I don't think he was used to girls he didn't have to work to get…or maybe he'd only seen me as part of the scenery. He was younger than me, and he probably saw me either as unattainable (best case scenario) or too old (worst case scenario). We went for a motorcycle ride later that week, and a few days later we went out to dinner. I paid, because I was the one who had asked him out. He appeared to be pleasantly surprised by my generosity.

It seemed only fair, but at the time I wasn't expecting it to become a pattern. I really didn't even think anything of it. I was just trying to be polite, and I desperately wanted to be liked. Since the motorcycle ride I had been unable to stop thinking about Jack. I like motorcycles, have owned several, and will probably own one again, but let's face it – the bike ride was just a cheap ploy to get my arms around him. I was lonely, and the more I thought about it I thought I once again needed the validation having a man in my life would bring me. Since it had been a while, I kept telling myself I was safe to try again. Never mind the fact that he wasn't interested in me until I asked him out. Never mind the fact that he'd been flirting with and hitting on every girl in the class for weeks – including Karyn, until he found out her age. He thought she was in her early 20s and was Max's girlfriend! It was just because he was lonely, I told myself. Once he got to know me he would want only me, and all his bad behavior would stop. I really thought that. I wonder now, in hindsight, just what kind of fantasy world I thought I was living in. It just goes to show that intelligence and common sense are far from one and the same. People are born with an intelligence level…common sense has to be learned – and very often it's learned the hard way.

About the time we got more serious, at least physically, another girl in the class became pregnant by a man who was also in the class – he was in the process of a divorce because his wife had caught him with the now-pregnant girl. That dojo was like my own personal soap opera. I loved going there, and I never knew what might happen next. There was always drama. I was proud that Karyn was doing well in the class, but mostly I was interested in seeing what kinds of things were happening next in the personal lives of the people. Pregnant-girl and almost-divorced-man decided they really did want to be with each other and they were going to stay together. Dojo love. I still couldn't tell you why, but I turned it into a competition. Everyone was talking about them – I wanted everyone to be talking about me! Pregnant-girl and almost-divorced-man were younger than me. She was also tinier, and cute and bubbly and giggly. Bubbly and giggly aren't terms most people would ever use to describe me. I'm usually very serious, and people mistake it for arrogance or snobbery. I wasn't feeling good about how much attention was being directed at them. *I* was supposed to be the star of the show. I started hanging all over Jack at every available opportunity, making how I felt very obvious to everyone. I put up with everything he did, and I laughed off anything that annoyed me or worried me, even when he got scary. His temper was legendary. He was all I talked about.

My parents got tired of it, my few friends (including my ex-husband Max) got tired of it, and everyone at the dojo got tired of it. The owner's wife even told me several times I was giving her *way* too much information. She started avoiding me. I knew I was doing it, but it was like I was powerless to quit. It really *was* an addiction in the truest sense of the word. I was desperate for people to talk to. Everyone *had* to know how happy I was, and how important I was because I had someone in my life. I craved their approval and their attention as a source of validation for myself. I talked about Jack *ad nauseum,* and I didn't seem to know how to stop, no matter how many people started rolling their eyes or suddenly realizing they had to be somewhere else *right then.* My mouth chattered on and on about this 'wonderful man' while the back of my brain desperately tried to kick my ass. He was unclean, uncouth, and uncivilized. He was also a lawbreaker and a troublemaker, with no regard for the people he harmed. Not to mention the lifestyle he was living would probably cause his death from alcohol poisoning, AIDS, or both before he reached a ripe old age. I told myself I wanted a wild, dangerous man like that. I told myself it was exciting. I'd been with the 'good guy' and had gotten bored. What better way to never be bored again? I worked every day to convince myself he was just what I wanted and needed. I never really did convince myself of it, but I told myself I had, and I went on seeing him.

One of my most serious problems was that once I started seeing someone, I didn't know how to break it off. I knew how to get divorced, but not how to stop having a boyfriend. Boyfriends led to fiancés led to husbands – I didn't understand that there could be an alternative concept. And now that pregnant-girl and almost-divorced-man were together, I tried everything I could to 'best' them. I was starting to see what a jerk I was dating, and there was already mounting evidence of some more serious control issues and anger management problems, but I couldn't possibly break up with Jack now. It would take me out of the competition and everyone would forget about me. I'd go back to being lonely and a loser and a nobody. It was ridiculous, I know. I saw that in the back of my mind, but I was completely incapable of stopping myself from carrying the relationship forward. Instead, in my mind it became a race between us and the other couple as to who could get the most serious in the quickest amount of time.

I doubt they were even aware they were running this race, because they didn't seem to have a need for those things. Unfortunately for me and my desire to get ahead of them and monopolize the limelight, they had a pregnancy going for them. I had no desire to get pregnant and Jack didn't want kids either, so that was out of the equation. I decided getting married, or at least getting engaged, would be the best option for me to be back in the spotlight at the dojo. In the process I could transform Jack into a good guy, and show everyone else how wrong they'd been about him. He would be my project, and I would make him into a great person, and we would live happily ever after. I *had* to do it, because I could see how everyone felt about us. How others felt about me always mattered to me then, even if I tried to pretend it didn't. They didn't really hide their contempt for Jack, and it was clear they thought I was just plain stupid. I'd show them. I wasn't going to let myself be looked at that way. I'd show everybody.

I started talking about marriage with Jack. I told him how much I liked being around him. I told him I loved him. He was quiet. Supposedly, he had some kind of fear about saying those three little words. I was willing to be patient.

"I feel it, but I just can't *say* it," he insisted.

I said it was all right. It didn't matter. *Of course it mattered!* But I was desperate to keep him. Losing him or dumping him would not only make me look like a failure, but it would get me a round of 'I-told-you-so's' that I didn't feel like listening to. I thought he might have some great potential locked up inside somewhere, even though he never failed to embarrass me at least once every time we were in public, was completely thoughtless regarding my money, space, possessions, or private time, and was merely tolerated by my parents. My father never said much about my choice in men, but I think he fervently hoped Jack might suffer some kind of tragic accident which would remove him from our immediate geographic area. My father's prayers were not to be answered.

Jack and I liked some of the same books and movies, and our senses of humor were actually quite similar. We probably would've been pretty good together in a relatively superficial friendship. I didn't really know how to be friends with a man, and it wasn't enough for me. A relationship was what defined me, and without a relationship I wasn't anyone. There was no sense of belonging. It wasn't long before we were spending all our free time together, and Karyn was doing everything she could to stay away from both of us. She never liked Jack. Sure, she thought he was funny sometimes, but beyond that she wanted nothing to do with him. I think she could sense something about him I was just blatantly ignoring.

Every day after school she would go straight next door to her grandparents' house and stay there, only coming home after dinner when she knew she didn't have a choice. She did this even if Jack wasn't there, telling me with her actions (had I been willing to acknowledge them) that she was upset with and disappointed in me, and that she really didn't want to be around me if I was willing to have a relationship with someone like

Jack. She probably figured saying something wouldn't make any difference, and at that time in my life she would've been right. I wasn't listening to anyone…not even myself. I'm sure Karyn felt trapped by her circumstances, too. Who wouldn't have? At that age, she couldn't live on her own. She could live with me or live with her father, and she wasn't seeing either one of those as great alternatives now that Jack was in the picture.

I, on the other hand, put up with amazing amounts of crap. Jack would say he was too busy to see me on a particular night, but then he'd call me up drunk at three or four in the morning and ask if he could come over. Apparently the bar scene wasn't working out for him or he was bored, or maybe he was just too drunk to know any better. Either way I always said 'of course,' and he would drive to my house and talk to me on his cell phone the entire way, right up until he pulled up in my driveway. While I was on the phone with him I was trying desperately to brush my teeth and hair, put on a better nightgown, etc., sometimes even hopping around on one foot, tripping over things, rather than stopping the conversation until he arrived. Why I didn't just hang up, I don't know. I guess I was afraid of hurting his feelings, especially if I told him he couldn't come over then – and if I didn't let him come to me when he'd been out drinking, I wasn't completely sure in the back of my mind if he might not go and seek solace in someone else's arms.

I told myself he must really care for me if he called me like that when he was supposed to be out having a good time with the guys. I was still half asleep, so I wasn't thinking clearly. I failed to see that what he was really trying to do was test me and see how much he could get away with – and how much I would put up with. He pulled stunts like that numerous times, and he would call me at least once a day yelling and cursing because he was allegedly being so badly mistreated at work. No one liked or understood him, he said, and although he did everything right, he was still treated badly. I had my suspicions about that, but I squashed them and tried to side with him, trying to be supportive as much as I was able. What he said *could* have been true – and I knew what it was like to be misunderstood and mistreated because you were different, since I had gone through it in school.

173

So I put up with the yelling and the cursing, and I put up with the lack of cleanliness and the lack of class. I put up with him rolling his eyes and telling me I just didn't understand when I didn't agree with everything he said. I put up with how *angry* he was – even when he was laughing. You could feel it there, just below the surface, and it's hard to thrive in an environment where there is so much negativity. I know he hated his job and people did make fun of him to some degree – that much was a fact, because I saw some of it firsthand on a couple of occasions. There were reasons for it, though, that I'm afraid he didn't see and I chose to deliberately ignore. He *made* himself a target for their harassment by being different – which is what I'd apparently done without realizing it all those years ago in elementary and middle school. I thought that fair was fair at that point, and maybe this was my purpose…to take someone who still had the same problems I used to have and 'fix' him. I wasn't happy with that idea, but I was trying to do what was right – or at least what I told myself was right. My ideas of right and wrong came from my parents, but they also came from what I wanted and felt that society wanted me to do. It made for a lot of confusion and angst, because I felt like I was being pulled in so many different directions all the time.

Even though we had a highly tumultuous and at times extremely volatile relationship, I talked more and more about marriage. Jack said very little, but he didn't seem to be that opposed to it. He mostly seemed indifferent, and I became almost frantically convinced I would lose him if I didn't marry him as soon as possible. I knew he had some problems. If I couldn't even keep a guy like Jack, what kind of a loser would I be then? I don't know why he married me. It might have been because he really did care about me. Then again, it might have been because of the equity line. I'd taken out a second mortgage on my house and was spending money left and right on things we wanted to do together and on things he wanted and needed. I also spent a lot of time looking around at different jewelry options, and I finally bought a wedding and engagement ring set online. It was the right size, and I took that as an omen that we were supposed to be together. I showed Jack some options for a man's wedding band and told him he could select whatever he wanted, and I would buy it for him. He picked the most expensive one, and I paid for all our rings with my credit card. Then I set a wedding date, insisting we get married before the year was out for the tax advantages it would give us. Have you noticed I didn't wait for something silly like an actual proposal? I never really asked him to marry me, and he never even came *close* to asking *me*. I just rolled right over the top of any objections he had to marriage and he eventually said I might as well go ahead and wear my engagement ring when it came in. And so I did.

I wore it to the dojo, and the pregnant girl saw it…and asked almost-divorced-man why *she* didn't have a ring on *her* finger. Oops. He had no good answer, only staring from me to the ring to pregnant-girl with a vacant, glazed expression normally seen on fish, and I secretly smirked on the inside. I had the spotlight back, and I was going to make the most of it. I acted so in love and so happy. When I was in private, I questioned just what the hell I thought I was doing. I knew, deep down, this guy was no good for me. It was that 'gut feeling' thing again – the one I'd been taught to ignore and repress. Even logically, marrying him didn't make any good sense at all. He was definitely not right for me. To this day, I still don't know if it was more that I thought I could 'fix' him or that I thought I didn't deserve any better. I'm at a loss to answer the questions that come with either one of those theories. I think it might have been some of both, depending on how I was feeling on any given day. The only thing I know for sure is I was glad pregnant-girl was jealous of me, but it wasn't long before she and her man got married. Almost right after his divorce was final, actually.

I remember my mother coming up to me about a month and a half before my wedding date and saying, "Well, she beat you. They got married at the courthouse yesterday."

She'd beaten me to the altar and it made me angry, depressed, and disappointed. They got a start on their new life before I did, and they had the limelight back. It wasn't fair. And then later that same night I comforted her and let her cry on my shoulder while her brand new husband wasn't paying attention because she wanted a 'real' wedding instead of the quickie courthouse one he had given her. She wasn't even given time to put makeup on or dress up, and it made her sad and ruined her special day. She was happy to be married, I guess, but still disappointed in the way the actual wedding had taken place. Seeing that, I couldn't be angry with her any more. I only felt bad for her, and her broken hopes and dreams. I wanted to make sure that didn't happen to Jack and me, and that we had a beautiful and magical wedding. I pictured charm and sophistication, and myself as the star of the show; all of the guests thinking how wonderful I was. Of course, that wasn't the way everything turned out.

I soon forgot about the issue of competition and focused completely on the wedding. I was the one paying. My parents had long since stopped paying for weddings (not that I blamed them) and for once I didn't even owe them any money they could write off for me as a wedding gift. I can't remember what kind of gift they got for us…it might have just been money…they may have paid for the cake. It all runs together in my mind, and some of my memories of my time with Jack are very sharp and clear, while others are really vague. I do remember the night Jack was kicked out of the dojo. He'd gotten his probationary black belt, but then the instructor decided he'd had enough, and he kicked him out. Of course I was incredibly angry. Looking back on it now I still honestly think it was unfair to let him get that far in his training and then deny him the right to attend for the next few months so he could complete his black belt. If the instructor was going to kick him out, he should have done it earlier on in the game. The problems he had with him hadn't just started. It's not that I think Jack was in the right with the way he often acted. It's just that I think the instructor did it deliberately to be cruel and show he had the power, and that still rankles me no matter what I think of Jack's attitude or actions. It also humbles me and makes me feel ashamed, because I've exercised power by being deliberately cruel in the past, and I now at least have more of a taste of what it feels like to be on the other end.

We got past the issue and finally everything was arranged for the wedding…flowers, cake, food, etc. The guest list had been adjusted to exclude the people from the dojo – Jack was still mad at them. He'd already moved all his things into my house months ago and we were getting married there, right in front of my fireplace in the living room, and then we were having the reception there as well. It was easy and convenient, and he didn't want to get married in a church. He wasn't of the Christian faith, instead opting for a more 'earthy' religion that believed in gods and goddesses, etc. I never saw him dance naked during the full moon or anything like that, but he definitely wasn't going to get married in a Christian church, and I definitely wasn't going to give up my religion. I might not actively *practice* it that much, but it was still mine. I still prayed and I still believed in God, even though I hadn't been back to church since Max and I parted ways. Occasionally I wondered if *God* still believed in *me*. We compromised on getting married at the house with a justice of the peace who promised to avoid all but one or two small references to Jesus. Jack said he could live with that and we went on from there, but it hurt my heart a little bit because the whole thing felt so Godless – no blessing on a marriage doesn't seem to be a great way to start one out. If I could have asked God, I'm not so sure He would have blessed that particular union anyway. I know no one else did.

In the last few days before the wedding actually took place I'd managed to yell at my mom, upset Karyn, irk my father, fight with Jack, and send Jack's mother – who I'd only just met – into a state of total piss-off because I paid for dinner one night. Not sure how anyone could get mad at someone else's generosity, but there you go. Maybe she took it for charity, which wasn't the case. Everything seemed to be going downhill as we got close to the big day. The wedding plans forged ahead despite everything that was going wrong in my life and everything that was pointing to this being a *very* dumb decision. It wasn't just Jack. It was me. It was Karyn. It was all of it. No one was happy, but we were trying to act like we were – like we were just putting on some kind of production, instead of living real life.

On the day of the wedding one of my friends came, along with two ex-husbands – Tyler (with his new wife) and Max – and my mom, dad, and daughter. The rest were people that Jack knew from his work. All in all there were only about fifteen of us. I don't think anyone was very interested in seeing him get married. No one liked him much. *I* didn't like him much.

Sad, but true. He hadn't changed at all in the brief time we'd dated, and despite my best efforts he was still a problem child. I was letting him ruin my relationship with my parents and my friends, and most importantly he was causing problems between Karyn and me. I should have gotten rid of him because of that, but I didn't. I was still so selfish and so convinced that I had started down this path and now I *had* to get something from it, no matter what the cost. I didn't actually *think* about sacrificing my own daughter to get what I wanted, but that was effectively what I was doing – and I didn't even really want him.

The day of my fifth wedding Karyn was ashen and silent, sick to her stomach and in real danger of passing out. My father left right after the ceremony, before the reception even started. He had walked me to Jack, but it was clear his heart wasn't in it. He looked like he wanted to be just about anywhere else. Tyler and his new wife kept exchanging *those* looks behind my back – you could see some of them in the wedding pictures before I threw them all away. The pictures weren't great – taken cheaply by an acquaintance who was actually a pretty good photographer most of the time, but for some reason didn't do very well that day. Maybe the unhappiness was seeping through. Before I walked from the back bedroom, down the hall, and over to where Jack was standing I almost threw up. I was upset, doubting myself, and knew I wasn't supposed to be doing this. I didn't want to go through with it and was already wishing I could back out, but I didn't see how that could happen.

All of the guests were there, and it was my house. It would have been hard to simply tell everyone I'd changed my mind and to get out…and what would Jack think? Would he be angry? Relieved? Sad? Bitter? Would he think I was joking or that I was crazy? Would he just leave, or would he want to try to work it out? What would my parents think after I'd spent all this money on Jack and the wedding and insisted I was happy, over and over again? My mother knew I wasn't really happy, because she saw how panicky and upset and depressed I was getting again. I was smoking heavily and drinking some and had lost weight. I didn't wear makeup any more or take care of myself. I felt lousy and frightened most of the time. It should have been a happy day, but I stood in that back room wishing I could just disappear and leave everything and everyone behind. Instead, I walked out there and said what I was supposed to say and we kissed and it was over and everyone moved into the dining room and kitchen to eat finger foods and cake and drink champagne and beer and soda.

Most of his friends got drunk and made a horrible, hellish mess in my kitchen. One of his bosses wanted me to go out back with him and get into the hot tub *and I thought about it*. He *was* really cute, after all, and his wife wasn't there that day. I wouldn't have really done it, but I was only a couple of hours into it and I was already unhappily married. I thought later I should have asked the lady who performed the ceremony to give me the marriage license she had signed. I could have just kept it and not turned it in to the courthouse, and the marriage wouldn't have technically existed. It would have been easier to get out of that way. Instead, I let her take it and turn it in. I was sick to my stomach most of the day and I had a golf ball-sized, infected, weeping sore on my body that I was trying to hide. Gross, I know, but true. It wasn't the first one, nor would it be the last, and I had gotten it because Jack was so unclean. He didn't even wash his hands after a bowel movement unless I yelled at him about it. He didn't shower much, and he often worked outdoors with his job, sometimes for days at a time. He was always scratching himself or had a finger in his nose or some other nasty place. Because he seemed to have some kind of crusade against personal hygiene he carried so much staph bacteria on his body, all over, that he was constantly getting boils and infections and MRSA, which is a drug-resistant staph infection that can be fatal if not quickly and properly treated. He was always at the doctor getting either oral or IV antibiotics, and then I started getting sick, too.

I'd had an old tattoo re-colored a few months before we got married and I thought the infection was from that, but it wasn't. I started having problems about a month after he moved in with me, and after he was gone I never had another problem, but I still carry a couple of scars from the infections. It could have gotten into my bloodstream, got to my heart, and killed me. But I was lucky, and I healed up OK. It isn't just relationship violence that can get you killed – sometimes it's things you wouldn't even think about or wouldn't even dream of. I had an open prescription for antibiotics from my dentist because of my prolapsed mitral valve. I was supposed to take meds before I had my teeth cleaned or other dental work done – the American Heart Association has since rescinded that requirement.

I filled the prescription again a couple days after the wedding and I took 2000 milligrams of antibiotic every day for 10 days straight, and I prayed I would be all right. I was sick, though, no question. I was shaky and feverish and had chills, and I wanted to sleep a lot. I didn't know which was worse: dying or having to live the way I was living. I didn't want to go to the doctor for something so humiliating and I didn't have any money, anyway. I'd spent it all on Jack and the wedding. The infection was in a bad place to show a stranger – very high up on the back of one thigh. I had so much pain in that leg for weeks that I could barely walk without wincing or crying out – it was hard to hide. I guess the infection ate into the muscle, too, because there's tissue damage there. Sometimes that leg still gives me trouble, but at least I'm alive and can get around. It could have been worse. I could have lost my leg...or my life.

I tried hard to actually love Jack instead of only saying I did. I really did try...but I just couldn't do it. It wasn't just the idea that I kept getting sick and wondering if it was going to kill me this time. Rather than tell Jack the truth I just tried to hide it, because I was ashamed to have these kinds of problems – even though they were caused by *his* unclean habits. No, it wasn't just that. It was everything. It was the way he stayed up until all hours, thoughtlessly keeping Karyn awake when she had school the next day because he apparently didn't come with a volume control. It was the way he drank himself to sleep a lot of nights, and farted on me and laughed about it. It was the way he shoveled in huge quantities of food and then complained he couldn't lose weight, and the way he spent all my money, including the equity line I'd taken out on my house.

Some of that was my fault...I didn't want to say 'no' to him, for fear he might leave and I would be alone yet again. And he was always yelling about one thing or another. Sometimes it was *to* me in a conversation about someone else. Sometimes it was *at* me. Oh, and then there was the way he called up other women and talked about how he couldn't wait to see them, and how much he wanted to 'do' the chick who had just cut his hair. Yes. I heard all of it, through our closed bedroom door. He talked so loudly I couldn't miss it. He thought I was outside but I wasn't, and I heard his 15 to 20 minute conversation with a lady-friend in another state. It wasn't pretty, and it wasn't nice for me to hear, but at least it made me aware. Something inside me rebelled. When he came out of the bedroom, I threw him out.

Karyn was glad to be rid of him. It was like a big weight had been lifted off her. I was miserable. Not because he was gone, but because I felt like I was failing again. We'd only been married a few weeks...what was I doing giving up on him already? Three days later he was back in my home after a very tearful meeting at a restaurant the day before. He explained to me he had some anger issues and other problems, and he didn't know marriage would be so difficult, and he didn't understand...didn't I care about him anymore? He sat and cried in a booth while people tried not to stare at this big guy sobbing, head in his hands, and this skinny, run-down-looking woman politely eating her sandwich. I still wasn't feeling very sympathetic. Did he genuinely care about me? Yes, I really think he did. If he didn't, I doubt he would've wanted to come back. Of course, it could have been the fact that he moved from a tiny, cramped, crappy apartment in an old building to a large, nearly-new house with land and money in the bank. Maybe in the end that was what he was crying over, and what he feared losing. I'll probably never really know, and ultimately it doesn't matter now.

I told myself he'd learned his lesson. I told myself he was sorry, and he didn't mean to hurt me, and he really did care about me. See how desperate I was to stay in a relationship? I was willing to put up with just about anything and forgive a lot of indiscretions to avoid what I perceived as the stink of failure. I was even willing to put up with the infections I kept getting...maybe eventually I would adjust to the high bacteria level and stop getting them, even thought he'd been getting them for years and it hadn't stopped yet. Maybe I'd be the lucky one. He came home and apologized to me, and to Karyn, and to my mother and father. He agreed to go to counseling for the issues he was dealing with, and he made appointments to do so. He actually even went a couple of times. I thought we were on the right track, and I was glad I'd given him another chance. I felt vindicated: see, I *can* fix this guy and make this work out!

A few short weeks later he did the same basic thing again. He clearly didn't care at all about anything that mattered to me. I guess it was just a game to him. You can't imagine how stupid I felt at that moment...or maybe some of you who are dealing with the same kinds of relationship problems – or have in the past – *can* imagine how stupid I felt. I found phone numbers I didn't recognize, women were calling him at late hours (he had conveniently forgotten to mention to them he had gotten married), *he* was the one who was usually too tired for sex or had some other excuse to avoid it, I found a lot of pornographic magazines – which I had asked him to please not bring to the house because I had a child there, I found hidden alcohol. I was always looking to see what else I could find. I was suspicious and a little paranoid by nature, mostly because of the way I was teased and harassed as a child at school mixed in with the problems with past marriages, and once a person had broken my trust it was very hard to get it back. He had broken my trust more than once. It didn't help that he wasn't the first husband to hide a passion for pornography from me or to talk about and/or go through with the idea of cheating. It made me a lot more sensitive to that part of the issue than I might have otherwise been.

After dealing with the latest round of drama and upset, I wasn't sure how much more I would be able to take. It seemed like it was too much to bear any longer. I was tired all the time – when I wasn't crying or panicking or letting my temper get the best of me. I thought I had needed a man to really *live*. Well, I *had* a man and I was back to just existing, with an existence that was markedly worse than before. I thought about throwing him out for a few days again to see if it would help, but I didn't think it would change anything. He wasn't making any effort I could see, and I wasn't willing to spend the next 10 or 15 years of my life waiting to see if that effort came to pass. I would be dead by then. My will to live would just be gone. I knew I hadn't been the perfect wife, but I felt completely undeserving of a user and a manipulator like Jack. No one should be treated that way, but I brought some of it on myself. I just wished I'd been willing to see him for what he was and acknowledge both his and my problems before we'd gotten married. It made me feel stupid, yet again. I came to a decision and knew he had to leave, but I wanted to be sure to be rid of him completely this time. I'd had enough, of both him and me.

The few shreds of dignity I had left after four failed marriages and a bankruptcy were shreds I wanted to keep, if there was any way I could. If I was able to just hold onto them, maybe someday I would be able to find a way to use them as a point to start rebuilding my life, such as it was. If it took a fifth failed marriage to keep that dignity, then so be it. Jack wasn't worth all of this. My panic attacks and depression had come back full force and were steadily getting worse instead of better, and of course he didn't understand or have sympathy with that. Mentally, I was a mess. I had trouble working and I just wanted to sleep to escape it all.

Physically I wasn't much better. Every time I had an itch I wondered if it was another infection getting started – often it was – and I wondered whether I would have to live my whole life this way. Karyn was a wreck, even worse than she was before. Her schoolwork was bad and her attitude of contempt and indifference to pretty much everything and everyone was even worse. I was worried she might even be suicidal, and I was afraid for her safety. I could hear her tossing and turning and grinding her teeth when she slept, and she never seemed to be rested. I noticed she occasionally had cuts and bruises on her that she couldn't explain. Had she done that to herself? I didn't know, but I was scared. It wasn't like I had some big revelation or something...I think I just became so tired of being sick and miserable that I was willing to do just about anything to stop it.

This time, I didn't really care if my parents looked down on me or not. I couldn't take this. I also didn't care whose fault it was any more. I just wanted it to be over with. I didn't even try to get him to walk out on me or anything. I didn't think I had the luxury of the time it would take for that to occur and the problems with his temper that might come about from it. I feared what he might do if the fighting escalated, and I feared what Karyn or I might do in retaliation. I already knew she was really beginning to loathe him. At times I thought she was just looking for some excuse she could use to justify hurting him – in self-defense, but possibly provoked.

With all of those things on my mind, I just plotted the best way to move him out of my life quickly and efficiently, with a minimum of fuss and bother. Over the course of a few days I made lists of the phone numbers I didn't recognize and copied the emails that were inappropriate. I printed out his profile from the dating sites. I kept track of any porn he viewed on either my computer or his. I took his wedding ring out of his gym bag. I took his house key off his key ring. He never noticed any of those things. He wasn't the most observant man in the world. I guess he thought I trusted him again, and that I was stupid enough to just go along with whatever he said he was doing or not doing. After all, I'd done it for this long, right? I didn't trust him at all. I don't know that I ever really had. I guess that's what happens when you marry someone you really don't know or even like that much, just so you can get married. What a waste.

The day after I liberated his house key he called me from work and I told him I knew about all the magazines and the Internet activity and the phone numbers. I told him he had betrayed my trust too many times and I wanted him out – it was over. He couldn't believe it. He thought I was crazy or joking, and finally came around to the realization that I wasn't either of those things. He was astounded I would divorce him over something he apparently saw as petty and unimportant. I don't know where he stayed that night. I didn't ask, and I didn't care. I spent the rest of the day systematically going through everything in my house, removing anything that belonged to him and making a pile in the middle of the floor of each room. It made a huge cluttered mess but I didn't care about that. I had an urge to drag it to the lawn and set fire to all of it, but jail time wasn't on my checklist. On the weekend he appeared with a truck and a few friends. They took boxes and garbage bags, filled them with his belongings, and he left. I sat on the couch with my mother, one of my pistols tucked into my waistband and concealed by my sweater, and waited until they all left. I didn't trust him, and didn't know what he might do. I didn't know if I was in danger or not, but I knew about his violent temper and anger management issues first hand, I knew he carried at least one weapon on him at virtually all times, and I wasn't taking any chances.

I wanted a divorce as soon as possible, and the fastest way to do that was for both of us to come to the filing and the hearing. Otherwise, it would drag out longer and become a lot more complicated. At least he complied and didn't make things any worse than they already were. I dreaded it, though. I worried about his mental state and my safety. I kept telling myself he wouldn't be allowed to carry a gun into the courthouse, but I slept badly for several nights and had dreams of him shooting me in cold blood rather than signing the papers, just because he thought I was an awful bitch and I had wronged him. During his tirades about people at work or on the highway or virtually anywhere else he often expressed himself with comments about how he was going to kill them or make them pay or other similar language. I never could tell with him if it was just macho talk or if he really meant it, but he certainly sounded like he wasn't joking. I wondered if I was on his list. Even though I didn't want to admit it because it made me feel like I was just being weak, I was afraid of him.

He met me at the courthouse on the day of our filing and again on the day of our proceedings, and we didn't have much to say to one another either time. After the judge signed the papers Jack walked out of the door with me and told me he was sorry it hadn't worked out. I said I was sorry as well, and I handed him a small packet with a few more of his things I had found around the house. He looked sad, and he looked like he might be about to hug me, so I stepped around him and walked quickly away, leaving with my mother and my aunt, who was in town visiting for a few days. She has now had the honor of being present at one of my weddings and one of my divorces. What a privilege for her, I'm sure. The three of us went out to lunch and talked about better things. I thought I might feel relieved, but I mostly just felt saddened and sickened by the whole mess, and wished that none of it had ever happened.

I pushed him into marriage. I know I did. I could see myself doing it while it was happening, but I couldn't seem to stop myself. A month after our wedding, for example, I made some comment about how I'd basically just said we were going

185

to get married, and he hadn't asked me. He told me that, had I been waiting for him to ask, I would still be waiting. I wanted to know why we got married, then. He shrugged. It'd seemed like a good idea to him at the time. I didn't know what to say to that, and after the divorce was final I didn't even know what direction to take with what was left of the rest of my life. I felt lost, and I wasn't sure how to get found again. Luckily for me God has a way of finding people, even when they don't know where they are…but first I had to go through a little more wilderness.

What I Did Wrong
- Turned marriage and love into a competition.
- Pressured someone who didn't love me into marrying me.
- Chose someone I wanted to 'fix,' and didn't back down even when it was clear that 'fixing' him wasn't possible.
- Went through with a wedding to a man I didn't even like by the time the wedding day rolled around, just so I wouldn't have to call it off and make myself look bad.
- Ignored how much my behavior was hurting my family – especially my daughter.
- Saw the cuts on my daughter's arms, knew in my heart she was hurting herself, and did nothing.
- Sacrificed my own physical and mental health because I didn't want to fail again, in my eyes or the eyes of others.
- Ignored my partner's serious problems (like anger management issues and lack of any kind of personal hygiene) just so I wouldn't be alone.

What To Look For
- Competing with others to keep the spotlight, get married first, have babies, etc.
- Trying to pressure or con or bribe someone into marrying you or staying with you.
- Not knowing when to say 'enough is enough' and end a relationship that you see is becoming more volatile.

- Going through with a wedding or any other kind of commitment to someone else just so people won't talk about you or so you won't look bad in front of others.
- Ignoring your own health and safety in order to stay with someone.
- Ignoring the needs of your family and friends, or ignoring changes in the behavior of your children.
- Seeing self-harming behaviors in yourself or a loved one and not doing anything about it because it's inconvenient or you don't want to deal with it.
- Overlooking serious relationship problems like anger, or a serious personal problem like unhygienic behavior that could make you very ill, just so you don't have to dump somebody and hear 'I told you so' from others.

What The Therapist Says

Before talking more about methods to ease the internal needs that cause codependent attitudes and resulting relationship addictions, we have to discuss a few concerns in this chapter that are too important to overlook. These concerns have to do with personal safety, or more precisely, the situations a relationship addict is liable to get into where his or her personal safety may be endangered. While everyone who has wound up in a relationship that turned dangerous has his or her own individual story, there are certain common patterns that can serve as warning signs.

Many times a relationship addict will begin to feel more confident about his or her ability to finally engage in a relationship that may work simply because a lot of time has elapsed since the last one. That is a false conclusion. As with many other addictions, temporary abstinence is not a cure. It does not even indicate betterment. If the addict does not engage in means to work on solving the internal issues that cause the addictive behavior the best that can be hoped for is that the state of the addiction does not become worse. Sadly, this is rarely the case. Many times the period of refraining from one's "drug of choice," in this case relationships, leads to a false sense of confidence that actually increases the likelihood of repeating previous behaviors and potentially repeating them on an even grander scale. Interestingly enough, the same pattern can be observed in more commonly recognized addictions such as alcoholism and drug abuse.

Warning signs that even a budding relationship has unhealthy components can be discovered simply by asking ourselves a few simple questions. The first one, strangely enough, would have to be, "How well do I know this person?" If the answer to this question includes a number of assumptions based on wishful thinking or past experience with other people the relationship may be headed for trouble. Concepts of the new partner fitting a certain "mold" of person that we are familiar with, of us assuming we know what this person must be "really" like underneath, those are things that do not bode well. The common factor is that the relationship addict assumes the new person of interest to be a certain way without actually knowing. Some people have called this fallacy the "mind-reading" concept, since the addict assumes he or she knows the intended's true self without having physical evidence of it.

The second question would have to be "Am I planning on changing my partner to improve him/her?" If one's hope for a happy-ever-after relationship is based heavily on the idea of changing, saving, or healing the partner in question then you have another warning sign that a severely unhealthy partnership is in the making. The idea that we have the power to change a person to become the ideal partner is as common in codependent thinking as it is dangerous. It is a simple fact that people who do not want to change are not liable to change, no matter how badly we want them to. If we engage in a relationship because we think that the right kind of kiss will turn our frog into Prince Charming we will wind up with only one thing: a very angry frog.

A common third question should be asked in situations where the relationship has already been initiated. This question can take four forms: (1) Am I willing to put up with awful behavior because I think he/she will change in the future? (2) Am I willing to put up with awful behavior because it is the best I will ever be able to get? (3) Am I willing to put up with awful behavior because it is my fault? Or the ever-popular (4) Am I willing to put up with awful behavior because now that I started a relationship I cannot get out? If the answer to any of these is yes than it is high time to re-evaluate how healthy or, more importantly, potentially dangerous the relationship might be. It is easy to see how a relationship addict may be willing to overlook undesirable, even risky behaviors in their partners due to any of these four ideas. Many an abusive relationship has been based and maintained on one or more of these four faulty assumptions.

The sad bottom line is this: a person's personal safety should not be compromised upon the ideas that love "might" be involved. If there are children involved this becomes even more important, as they are even more helpless to potential abuse by partners who exhibit dangerous behaviors but are tolerated because of codependent beliefs. This chapter is the best example of why it is essential for anyone with codependent attitudes and relationship addiction to take the time and face the issues that cause them. Only by facing them, understanding them, and then working on healing them can potentially hazardous relationship scenarios be escaped from before they become too dangerous.

We have already started talking about how the subconscious mind works and how it comes to believe in codependent ideas. We know what we learn about the world and ourselves comes, in large part, from what we see mirrored in our families and peers. While the first step then is to understand what motivates our low self-esteem and the overall feeling that we need outside approval and attention to feel worthwhile, it requires more than an understanding of why we act the way we do as far as relationships are concerned. In the beginning of the healing process the first thing to learn is probably one of the most difficult. Whenever a relationship addict feels attracted to a new partner, especially early in recovery, he or she must "stop and think" rather than simply act on impulse. A lot of times our codependent needs lead us to act rashly and quickly, seeking immediate gratification to whatever our codependent need may be at the time. Learning to stop rather than reacting immediately can be a lifesaver.

This is not an easy thing to do. Actually, it is a very uncomfortable thing to do because it keeps us from what we really want at the moment, which is to be with that person. But the simple fact that we so desperately seem to need that new partnership is a good warning sign for us to take a mental step back and identify our own motives. Thoughts that help in this "stop everything for a moment" idea can include motivators like: "Let me think this over. I want to get it right this time." If the relationship addict feels a sense of having to act immediately because of the relationship "opportunity" potentially slipping away assurances like: "I have time to get this right" may also be of help. Any rational thought that validates taking the time out to understand what makes us want to engage in a relationship can be used that way. Note that we do not even have to believe these thoughts. Simply allowing ourselves to engage in these thoughts can give us a short bit of breathing space that can allow us to investigate our motivation.

Once a codependent has managed to take this mental "time out" the difficult questions arise, the ones we all fear to entertain because of the answers they may yield. The simplest form of these would be: "Why do I want this relationship?" And the answer to this question, since it is asked in relation to our own attitudes, should reflect those attitudes. If at any point the answers to this include such ideas as: "I do not want to be alone anymore," "I need him/her," or "I feel incomplete without this" then the relationship in question would appear to have its roots in our codependent needs rather than love. This is a good indicator that we are about to engage in our old addictive habits again, no matter how desperately we want to believe that this time it is different. Actually, the aspect of desperation in our motives is probably the very best indicator that what we are about to engage in is founded in addiction rather than love. If this desperation is present then the codependent individual in question should refrain from taking the relationship any further.

Of course, at this point the question of how one can distinguish real love from addictive love has to come up. It may be a frightening prospect for a relationship addict to realize that he or she never experienced any relationship without this facet of need and desperation. The individual in question may fear that he or she never actually knew love without these attached facets. The addict might even worry that he or she is incapable of true, non-addictive love since it is such an unknown. These fears are understandable, but thankfully invalid. Just because we do not know something or have not learned it yet, does not mean we cannot learn it at all. After all, the codependency that is at the root of most relationship addiction is a learned habit of thought and action. Therefore healthier forms of love can be learned as well, if we are willing to make the effort. Once we are willing to take the first step, which is realizing our addictive patterns and then taking a stance to stop whenever we fear we may re-engage in the old patterns, we can begin learning about healthy, true love.

Chapter 8: Anxiety, Depression, and Self-Worth

It's important here to take a break from my relationship history, for two reasons. First, because the last chapter marked the end of the marriages (but definitely not the end of the story) and second because it's necessary to address my state of mind at that point in time. It'll give you a better understanding of how this was taking its toll. Relationship addiction can wear you down, make you feel worthless and stupid, and make you wonder just what in the world is *wrong* with you that you can't seem to be happy with yourself or anyone else. In that way, I would say it's very similar to other types of addictions, such as those to drugs or alcohol. Some part of you, on some level, *knows* what you're doing is wrong, but you find so many ways to justify it and overlook the problems with it that you basically convince yourself you're doing things right and it's the rest of the world that's screwed up. I really do think sometimes this world *is* screwed up in many ways, but that doesn't mean *I* have to be, or that I should take the 'It's OK because everyone else is doing it' attitude.

I remember crying on my parents' shoulders and the shoulders of my few remaining friends both during my marriage to Jack and after it was over, asking why this happened; not yet understanding I was the one causing this. Not anyone else, but me. Granted, the men I chose throughout my life might have been all wrong for me, and some of them were definitely not the best of people, for various reasons. But that wasn't what ultimately mattered. What mattered was *I was the one who kept choosing them.* I should have walked away but I didn't seem to be able to, and look how much misery it had led me to. I didn't think I mattered any more. How could anyone care about me? How could my parents and family still love me? How could *God* still love me? Surely everyone had given up on me by now. I was so ashamed I basically just stopped caring about everything. I stopped living and went back to existing. It was easier than trying to pretend things would get better, and it felt safer. Since I didn't feel like I had any worth left or any value to society I slept a lot, I worked only enough to pay my bills, and I only did what I absolutely *had* to do for those around me, including Karyn. I hated my life, because I hated myself. Those 'shreds of dignity' I'd wanted to hold onto had disappeared somewhere. I didn't recall misplacing them or giving them away, but I couldn't seem to locate them anywhere.

If you've ever had depression or known someone who has, you know it isn't always pretty, and there are really no quick fixes. You also know that it's a battle not everyone wins. A lot of depressed people take their own lives because they can't see anything better for their future, or they don't want to try again, or for similar reasons. Life simply becomes too much for them. The same is true for any kind of panic or anxiety disorder, and the same is true for a lack of self-worth. All those things wear you down until you get to the point where you feel like life really *isn't* worth living any more. I can talk about it more easily now, because a little time has passed since I've been there. The time during my fifth marriage and after it ended was the worst time in my life. While there were a lot of bad moments throughout my childhood and early adulthood, they weren't as prolonged and as devastating as the point I had reached in early 2006. I was tired all the time, and I didn't want to do anything. Even going to the store or doing laundry was becoming too great a task for me to complete with any frequency. I had no desire to take good care of myself, I ate very little and was looking almost skeletal, and I had no real interest in trying to make my life better. Who cared?

Add to that the fact I was very often angry, and I continued to have panic attacks on a daily basis, sometimes having one that would literally last for hours. Some doctors will tell you a panic attack cannot sustain itself for more than 20 minutes or so. They are wrong. I was depressed, anxious, and suffering from a lack of concern for much of anything, no question, but that wasn't the worst of the issue. What was worse was that I began to see these traits coming out more and more clearly in my daughter. She'd been dragged through 'stepfathers on parade' for many years, and it had taken its toll on her, as well. She no longer trusted anyone, including me. At thirteen she was overweight, didn't take care of herself, and didn't care to change that. Her hair was frizzy and her skin was bad, and I imagine she felt like she was ugly and wasn't worth a whole lot to anyone.

She certainly *acted* like she felt that way, but she wouldn't talk about it. She had no friends, was being teased in school relentlessly each day, and her schoolwork was mediocre, even though I knew she was very intelligent. It wasn't that she couldn't do the work, but she was so unhappy she didn't pay attention and couldn't concentrate. She just wanted to be left alone, but of course the curse of people who just want to be left alone and not be a bother to anyone is that no one leaves them alone and everyone bothers them. She started getting headaches all the time. Almost every day she'd come home with a headache, and she just wanted to lie on her bed in her darkened bedroom and be left alone. I didn't know what to do with her.

There were a few good days, but not too many. Both of us were spiraling downward, and even if I'd known how to stop it, I doubt I would've cared enough about either one of us at that time to do so. What did it matter anyway? She'd be better off without me. I'd ruined so much of her young life already, and I figured I was just going to make it worse in the future. Again my thoughts turned to suicide, but I never tried it. I was afraid of what might come next, afraid I would go to Hell, afraid of what it might do to my parents. I was always afraid of something, either real or imagined. At least I had my house back, along with my peace and quiet, but it was a hollow victory. I went through periods of being so grateful Jack was gone, and other periods of thinking I should have tried to work it out so I wouldn't be alone. I couldn't decide which was worse, and there were even a few times where I almost called him or emailed him, but I stopped myself before I could actually go through with it. What would it have solved?

I was sure he'd moved on and had no further interest in me. If he'd really cared, he would've fought to keep the marriage instead of just letting it go. I think that was one of the things that bothered me the most. Just because I didn't still want *him* didn't mean he wasn't supposed to still want *me*. I'd given him so much, I thought, while we were together, and then he just walked away when I said I wanted out because of his transgressions. He didn't beg or plead. He didn't try to stop me. He just said OK and left.

Not even being worth the attention of someone you think is a real loser is depressing. I tried telling myself he didn't know what he was missing and I was just way too good for him, but when you're depressed and you try to think those thoughts your mind just says, 'Yeah, right. And what makes *you* so special?' and you're right back to being depressed again. Sometimes trying to think positively during that time in my life even made me feel worse, because I felt like I was getting my hopes up only to have them stepped on, again and again. I didn't feel like I had a *right* to think positively, or to have anything good in my life again. Efforts by my parents and friends to help me feel better made little headway. This was something I would have to do on my own, when and if I ever decided I wanted to, or ever found a reason to. For months I just didn't care. I was going through the motions of living, but I didn't feel much of anything really, except for sadness and self-loathing and fear. All the 'good' emotions – all the laughter and the happiness and the joy – were basically alien concepts to me. I'd forgotten what most of them felt like. Karyn was pretty much the same, but I didn't notice it that much. We were both so busy with our own misery we weren't bothering to look at anyone else's. Life became a matter of getting through each day, only to get up and do it all again the next day.

The only reason I finally got so tired of feeling bad that I forced myself to go to a local clinic and see about getting medicated for my problems was that I got bored and angry. I lost my temper. I was bored with feeling miserable, because there was really no drama in it. After a while your friends just stop talking to you much and your parents get tired of trying to make you feel better because you won't try to help yourself. You don't have much, and you get tired of the fact that nothing is changing. I laid around for months, barely getting by and saying, 'oh, poor me, poor me,' and getting more and more upset that no one was coming along to rescue me and make me feel better. I had been through so much...why should *I* have to work to feel better? Shouldn't someone else do that for me? I went back and forth between thinking I wasn't worth saving and thinking the world *owed* me for all the pain I had already suffered. Wasn't God supposed to be merciful? Where was my mercy? Or maybe God was tired of me, too. I was definitely tired of myself, and it seemed like pretty much everyone around me was tired of me as well, so I guess God might as well join the group.

I'd gone out to the yard one day because it was overgrown and needed work, and I sat in what was left of the grass and listlessly started pulling some weeds. I didn't have much enthusiasm for the task, but it was the first time in months I'd even felt like doing anything at all. The yard reminded me of my life…it used to be pretty but now it was aging and neglected, and no one really gave it a second glance any more – not even its owner. Maybe it would make me feel better if the yard looked better. Who knew? It was worth a try, but after looking around it also seemed like a very prolonged and maybe even impossible task. Still, I tugged away at sticker vines and other intruders. I'd only pulled a few weeds when pain shot up my left arm and into my chest, sending me into a huge panic attack. I was so tired of these damn things! Weren't they *ever* going to go *away*? They used to go into remission after being around for a year or so, but it'd been almost two years since they'd returned, and they were getting worse instead of better. To top that off, all the chest pain I was getting made me seriously concerned – again – that there actually *was* something wrong with my heart. Just because I hadn't dropped dead didn't mean I wasn't about to. I lived my life in fear of my death, every day…and I didn't even have a husband who would mourn me. How pathetic I must seem to others, and how pathetic I seemed to myself.

I sat in the yard and threw a tantrum. I did. There's just no nice way to say it. I threw my gloves and pounded my fists on the ground and yelled and kicked and screamed, tears streaming down my face. I was *tired!* Tired of all of it. Tired of feeling second-class. Tired of feeling afraid. Tired of not having any money. Tired of feeling like I wasn't worthwhile. Tired of myself. I *wanted* to be worthwhile. That little spark was still alive, deep down in my soul. I wanted to matter for the right reasons, but I didn't know how. When I was done with my fit I was still panicky, but I was also still angry. I got up and found an address for a local urgent-care clinic where I didn't need an appointment, and I got in my car. I told my parents where I was going and why and they said to drive carefully, and I left. Going to the doctor was a huge step for me, because anyone who knows me will tell you I am seriously afraid of doctors and I *hate* taking medication. It's a battle to get me to take an aspirin for a headache. I loathe it, because I'm always afraid it's going to do something horrible to me or kill me.

The doctor at the local clinic was unimpressed with my self-diagnosis of mitral valve prolapse syndrome. He insisted it was all in my head – a little woman like me shouldn't be surprised to be overwhelmed by the big ol' world – and he gave me a prescription drug designed to treat anxiety and depression. He said he thought he might be able to hear a faint heart murmur but wasn't sure, and I should get it checked out when I could afford it – I didn't need to do it right now, and it probably wasn't serious. That should have made me feel better, but for some reason it didn't. I think it was mostly his attitude and the careless way he dealt with my problems. It was the 'good ol' boy' network of health care, one of the curses of many places in the south. It furthered my belief that I was unimportant and didn't really matter. Even though I'd sensed that the little spark was still there when I'd had my temper tantrum in my front yard, there used to be a roaring flame in me that kept saying I *did* matter and I *was* worthy of better than this. I'd *burned* with life when I was younger, despite the problems I'd had. I'd been through so much that now it had been reduced to that tiny, glowing ember. I wondered from time to time why it was even still there at all, and what would happen if it went out. Would I die? I didn't know. And I didn't remember how to fan that little ember anymore and make a flame again. I had long since forgotten.

Handing me the trial package of medication, the doctor told me to take one pill per day and to *not*, under *any circumstances,* read the listed side effects on the package or look them up on the Internet. Don't research it. For Heaven's sake don't Google it! I'd just scare myself. Just take the medication and come back to see him in two weeks when it was almost gone so that he could raise the dosage. This was only 12.5 mg – a starter dosage that would need to be increased, probably several times, to reach a therapeutic dosage of 50 mg or so, perhaps more. A medical doctor who forbade his patients to read pertinent information that they might need for their own safety because he didn't take their problems seriously? This is where health care has gotten to in so many places throughout this country. No wonder there are problems. But I took the pills home and called my parents on the way to let them know what was said. My mom and dad must not have thought there was really anything seriously wrong with me or they would have driven me to the doctor, instead of letting me make the 20-minute commute on my own and sit alone in the waiting room for hours, wondering what would happen. I wasn't sure whether to be pleased they had faith in me or angry they weren't concerned enough to insist they should come along. I wanted the comfort, but I didn't want to be seen as weak – I think my dad had seen me that way enough times already, but that could've just been my own perception.

I hadn't eaten all day…I felt too bad and when I was anxious the first thing that stopped was my food intake. I ate very little dinner when I got home from the clinic, and I took my first pill before I went to bed. I felt pretty good for the first time that day, so I was cautiously optimistic. I woke up about three or four times during the night to use the restroom, which wasn't normal for me. Once I almost fell, and twice I walked into the wall. *That* wasn't normal for me, either. I was always one of those 'instantly awake' people who could go from 0 to 60 in just a couple of seconds. Sleep didn't cling to me and make me bump into things. I was too tired and dizzy to think much about it overnight, other than to think it was odd. I wasn't even coherent enough to be afraid, but when I woke up in the morning I was in a fully fledged panic attack – one far, far worse than I'd ever had before. It was so bad I literally couldn't sit still. In order to keep me in a chair I would have had to have been physically restrained. I woke Karyn and we went to my parents' house, where I proceeded to completely lose it for a few hours. I couldn't stop crying, and I remember hugging my mother in the kitchen, begging her over and over again to please not let me die. Later I walked lap after lap around her dining room table, still crying, clenching and unclenching my fists – anything to keep moving. Yet I was exhausted, both physically and mentally.

I called the doctor's office and the nurse said to take Benadryl to counteract 'the jitters.' I asked for something stronger and was refused. They weren't exactly taking me seriously…I felt like they thought I was weak, and I was taking a little reaction and blowing it out of proportion, but I wasn't. I liked drama in my life, but this was the kind of drama I would gladly do without. I really felt as though I might die if my heart kept racing like it was. My mom brought me some Benadryl but one of the side effects listed on the box was anxiety, so I passed on that and just rode it out. Why try to make it worse? When I finally felt like I could stop moving I spent most of the late afternoon huddled on the floor in my mom's office while Karyn watched over me with something approaching real concern and I tried desperately to distract myself with television. My heart had been pounding for hours and I was cold and frightened and shaking. I tried calling the doctor again but wasn't given any help, even though the list of side effects clearly said to call your doctor if you were having the kinds of problems I was having. They just told me to skip that night's pill and take the next one in the morning, and eat more. No one seemed to care that much, but I guess there really was little they could do. I would just have to wait until my system processed the medication and hopefully got rid of it quickly.

I started thinking about medication while I was lying there, staring mindlessly at the television and feeling sorry for myself. When I'd been in hard labor with Karyn I'd been given pain medication that was only supposed to make me doze between contractions and wake up during them so I could get a little bit of relief. I was out cold for over half an hour from only 1mg of the drug. I didn't feel a single contraction, and when I woke up it was time to push and Karyn was born only half an hour later, so these weren't just little, easily ignored cramps. These were the real deal. I guess I was still overly sensitive to medication, and the anti-anxiety meds were no exception to that particular rule. Thinking of that added to my panic and despair. I was sick and panicky and miserable, *and there was nothing I could take to help me.* Late that night when I finally started to feel a little better I flushed the rest of the medication down the toilet and decided I would never again take anything for anxiety or depression. There were other drugs I could've tried, but it wasn't worth it to me. If I had to go through weeks of that just to see if the medication would work I feared I might *really* consider suicide. I don't think I could have lived with that level of sheer terror for much longer. There had to be a better way for me.

That emphatically doesn't mean I'm against medication for anxiety and depression, or for any other physical or mental problem. Most people can take those kinds of medications with minimal side effects. I think people should use what works for them, as long as it's legal, safe and effective, and as long as it's used responsibly. I recovered from that medication episode slowly, and I lost what little faith I still had in the medical community in my geographical area. I'm sure there are many, many good doctors out there throughout the world today. Unfortunately, I've had poor and upsetting experiences in trying to find them and have mostly given up on that idea. When my time comes I'll have to die inefficiently, without their help. I've found, at least for me, that they don't seem to take problems seriously, and they really don't have 'cures' for most of the problems human beings develop.

The same is true with problems like relationship addiction. You can't 'cure' it, but you *can* understand and be aware of it, and you *can* learn to make better choices – and that will help you to start feeling better. Most of your ability to help yourself comes from a conscious effort to do so, coupled with a lot of work. Not everyone wants to do this kind of work; for a long time I didn't want to, either. I wanted someone else to do it for me. I wanted the rewards, and I wanted them *now,* but I just wanted them handed to me – I didn't actually want to *work* for them. It seemed like too much effort and like it would take way too long. It's not something that can be done overnight and it's not something someone else can do for you. In addition, you have to be *aware* of what's going on, and you have to acknowledge it. That can be extremely difficult, and it's the part of the problem I struggled with the most. It took me a long time to feel truly better on a consistent basis and to see that the trail of destruction I'd left in my life was mostly self-caused. I could've picked the best man in the world the first time out...or any time out, but it would've ended up the same. Despite their flaws and the problems we had it really wasn't them...it was me. All me.

I don't mean to say I deserved to be treated poorly, or I should have been abused, raped, or cheated on. What I mean by saying it was all me is that I was the one who needed the help to break the pattern and find the kind of life I really should have been living. I was the one who should have made my own choices, instead of only living my life the way I thought others wanted me to, or feeling as though I couldn't be anyone if I were on my own. To some extent what caused me to take the path I took is still a mystery. It's hard to say how these things get started, and there are a lot of different triggers. Part of it was my childhood, I'm sure – from my desire to always please my parents to the way I was teased and abused at school, but I seriously doubt that was all of it. A lot of people go through similar things with childhood teasing and all, and they turn out 'normal.' Some of it is probably genetic makeup as well. Just like some people are predisposed to cancer or heart disease, some people are predisposed to anxiety, depression, and addictive behaviors. Surely you've heard people say a certain person 'has an addictive personality'? So why does that addiction always have to be about alcohol or drugs? The truth is that it doesn't. People can become addicted to anything, and for all sorts of reasons.

While I struggled through my addiction to relationships and love, there were people all around me – some who I came into contact with and some who I didn't – who were addicted to drugs, alcohol, fetishes, and all sorts of things. Even becoming a recluse because you want to stay home all day and build model ships, for example, is an addiction. Whether it's unhealthy or not depends a lot on whether you still bathe and go to work and have a life outside of it or whether it consumes you. With me, the idea of a relationship consumed me. I *had* to have one, and I *had* to have the approval of others. This often put me in the spotlight, which you'd think I would hate since I was so shy as a child, but I lived for the praise. The spotlight was welcome because it made me feel like I had importance to someone besides myself. That whole idea of 'mattering' was highly significant to me, but somewhere along the line I became too focused on mattering to others and forgot that who I was and what I did ultimately needed to matter to myself. If that hadn't been the case things might have turned out quite differently, but that's something I'll never know in this life.

Self-worth – that sense of mattering – plays a large part when it comes to a person's addiction, in two different ways. Having a lack of self-worth can cause a person to involve himself or herself in addictive behaviors, but conversely, having an addictive behavior can also harm a person's self-worth. You see the problem? It's a double-edged sword, and one that can spiral out of control, often quickly and before a person has a chance to stop and realize what's going on. By the time a person sees that there's a problem, it can be so deeply entrenched that it's hard to break and takes a lot of work, and that's the *good* news. The bad news is that for many people there's never any realization at all, and because of that they never get the chance to break their addiction or improve their quality of life. These are the people who end up dead, or who spend their days wishing they were. They may see jail time if their addiction is to drugs or alcohol, they may get behind the wheel and kill someone, or they may abuse their children or their spouse. I should be – and I am – grateful that those addictions are not my addiction. Having said that, relationship addiction can be, in some ways, harder to treat.

There is no detox center you can check yourself into when you have this kind of problem. No intervention program where you are re-trained to be alone and enjoy it. There are groups and organizations that can be of help and information on those, as well as books, articles, and websites, can be found in chapter twelve, but these are not the same as an inpatient style of treatment. If there are any inpatient opportunities for relationship addiction within the United States or other well-developed countries, I'm not aware of them. Relationship addiction must be approached differently, but like other types of addictions the addicted person must at some point take responsibility for his or her own actions, and 'own up' if you will to what took place in the past. If you're struggling with depression and/or anxiety on top of addiction, like I was, it becomes even more difficult to come to this acceptance. This is the one step a lot of people never take. It took me the longest, and it honestly happened mostly by accident. I wasn't expecting it, and I didn't even see it coming – sometimes we get blindsided in a good way. It doesn't happen very often but when it does we can be sure there's a reason for it.

My parents always used to tell me that time had a way of working things out, and I'd always roll my eyes when they said that. I thought it was just one of those things parents said. Whatever was wrong, I wanted it fixed right then. As I get older, I notice things do seem to work out if I'm patient with them while still doing what I can to help them along. It's amazing the wisdom you sometimes find as you get a little older. My daughter is very fortunate to have acquired that understanding almost from birth, but it's not something that's common in a young person. I don't even see it in too many older people today, which is unfortunate. With a problem like relationship addiction, it's even harder to see that things will work out if you're patient with them while still moving toward getting help. You don't want to take a deep breath and see what you really *need to* do next. Instead, you're always looking for that next person, that next love, that next little bit of drama to make you feel important and to make your life complete. When it doesn't appear on your terms you go hunting for it, trying to force the universe to conform to your idea of what's right. It usually backfires.

I hadn't seen the problems I was having while I was right in the middle of them. Who does? Oh, I knew something was wrong. I just refused to acknowledge it and admit it was *my* problem and not a problem with someone else or with society as a whole. By the time I came around to the idea that I wasn't doing well running my life the way I'd been, I'd already made a pretty serious mess of it over a lot of years. Even with that realization I certainly hadn't moved to the outside of the mess, but I was closer to the edge than the middle and I could begin to see some of the issues I'd created in my life. It hurt me to see they weren't just my problems but my daughter's problems as well. I didn't want her to grow up unhappy, and I knew I had to change to help her. By the time I reached the lowest point in my life she was already in her early teens, and struggling. I had higher hopes for her than where her life was going. Who doesn't want more for their child than what they had? I'd had all the basic comforts as a child, and I'd enjoyed some things most kids don't get like family vacations and parents who clearly wanted me to have the best in life, even if they didn't always go about it the right way. Parenting by myself was hard, and parading men through our lives wasn't making it any easier for a young and impressionable girl.

The problem I was having with Karyn was that I wasn't sure how to approach the issue. I knew her trust in me when I said 'no more stepfathers' was seriously lacking. I'd said it before, and it hadn't come true. How was she supposed to believe me? I was willing to let her be mistrustful...there wasn't much I was able to do about that. What I *could* do was start to show her there was more to life than the kinds of things she'd experienced. I wanted to do that, and I felt she needed that, but I didn't really have any idea how I could go about it. What would work, and what would be useless? How long would it take? How much effort would I have to put into it? I was still depressed and anxious, and I was still feeling unimportant. Just one more insignificant speck of a human on an insignificant speck of a planet, hurtling through space for an unknown purpose. I had to get myself out of my depression and I had to get my anxiety under control, but those kinds of things were easier said than done. And of course I was lonely. There was no man in my life, and there was no drama in it. How had I managed to get to this point?

Ironically, I hadn't yet realized that I got upset with boredom and went looking for drama, then got upset at the drama and went looking for boredom. That was the story of my life; something I'd always done and always failed to acknowledge. If I'd seen that pattern years ago I wonder what my life would have been like. I don't know and can't even really speculate, but I'll bet it would have been different...or maybe not. Maybe I would have done the same things and just been more aware of them, making me feel like an even bigger fool. Sometimes ignorance is bliss. I'd finally reached a point where I really, honestly wanted to change. That was the key. I *wanted* to change. I wasn't happy with myself and I hadn't been happy with me for as long as I could remember. Having some happy moments or having some accomplishments is not the same as really being happy with who you are on the inside. I was ready to find that happiness, but there was a catch. I didn't know how to do it, and I didn't want to really have to work for it. I still secretly hoped someone would just hand it over to me, so I waited a while longer. Nothing happened. Finally, I decided my greatest accomplishment and the source of my happiness would come from solving my problems – the anxiety and depression I had – myself. I still didn't know I was 'officially' a relationship addict. I'd still never heard the term and didn't know what it meant. If you would've told me then that I was an addict, I would've looked at you like you'd gone crazy. I rarely drank at all anymore and I didn't ever do drugs…how could I be an addict? I still wasn't ready or willing to acknowledge that sort of thing in my life.

I reasoned the depression came from the anxiety. If I could stop panicking, maybe I could stop feeling so down about myself. I wouldn't be as afraid to do anything, and perhaps I could get some exercise, get in better shape, and boost my self-esteem. I knew I needed the exercise, because the lack of it was contributing to my chest pain. It was the muscles that were causing the problem. I didn't use them much, so when I did need them for something they responded by hurting and aching and twanging – pains that I took, in my over-sensitive state, for 'chest pains' related to a heart problem. It made sense, and I knew using my muscles was the only way to correct the problem. It seemed like a plan, but I wasn't exactly convinced I could stop panicking. In the past I'd tried all kinds of things, and nothing worked completely. Even thinking about exercising or moving around much had me vaguely nervous. I didn't hold out a lot of hope I'd be able to find a solution. For the first time in a long time, I wanted to try. It was time to do something new, and I kept feeling like I wanted to change and I *needed* to change.

In an effort to find inspiration and help and confidence I started praying more, but I wasn't sure I was getting a whole lot out of it. I didn't really feel forgiven, and forgiveness is one of those things you either believe you have or believe you don't have. There is no tangible, proven way to see whether you've got it or not. It's all about faith. Prayer had become only repetition to me. In my head, before I went to sleep each night, I said the words I had been taught to say through going to church with Max. There was little feeling being put into it, which was probably why I wasn't getting much out of it. I tried to encourage Karyn to pray as well, but she had the same problem I did. It wasn't that she didn't believe, but that we'd both forgotten how to *talk to* the God we believed in.

If you're getting uncomfortable with this because you're not Christian, please don't let that bother you. It doesn't matter to me whether you believe in the same God I do. That's not the point of this. The point is that *whatever* you believe in…regardless of what you call that higher power…connecting with Him/Her/It can help you and bring you some peace. I thought it was easy, but it's not. Just saying words you think you should be saying won't do it. It really does have to come from your heart…and some people don't have a higher power they believe in. If you're one of them, there must be something that matters to you or that you have a reverence for. Maybe it's nature, or perhaps it's something else entirely. Whatever it is, you can use it to help make yourself feel more connected. I don't mean you should go out and pray to a tree, but you can use the enjoyment you get from the nature all around you, or whatever works for you as a focal point, as a way to feel more connected to the rest of the world, and as a way to realize that all things, great and small, have meaning, value, and importance beyond measure – including you and me.

Since I wasn't getting that feeling from praying before I fell asleep, I knew there was something else I should be doing instead, but I wasn't sure what it was. That traditional style of conservative Christianity was all I knew, and all I had taught to Karyn. I felt like anything outside those lines was somehow blasphemous or wrong. I remember being shocked and appalled when a girl I went to college with during my time with Max said when she addressed God in her prayers, she called Him 'Daddy.' It seemed so…so *irreverent.* I didn't seem to be able to feel any connection with God, and I hadn't done very well at connecting with people, either. I'd already made it into my mid-thirties, and all I had to show for it was five failed marriages, a strained relationship with my parents, no real, true friends outside of ex-husbands and family members, and a daughter who seemed to want little to do with me – and little to do with herself. Obviously my ability to connect with anything or anyone was seriously questionable, and that was depressing, no matter what else I was thinking about when it came to wanting and needing a change. Could I learn to connect? I didn't know. Would it really help? I didn't know that, either. It kept nagging at me, running around and around in the back of my mind. It wouldn't let me rest, even if I tried to ignore it.

I thought about giving up on all of it, but I couldn't shake that overwhelming feeling that it was time for a change. I'm sure you know what it's like to have a thought pester you. Maybe it's a song you can't get out of your head, or something you think you've forgotten at the store. Thoughts can nag us no matter what else is going on. Some thoughts, though…some thoughts pester us so much and are so significant to us we know we must do something with them, even if we don't want to. Even if we don't know how to. Even if we are afraid. No matter how depressed I tried to stay, those nagging thoughts of change just wouldn't leave me. Yes, I did say 'how depressed I *tried* to stay.' It's true. I actively *tried* to remain depressed and miserable for weeks, because I was too afraid of what would come next. I was afraid of the idea of trying to change anything for the better. Which is safer – the devil you know, or the devil you don't know? I just couldn't see how I could do anything differently. I couldn't change the past, and I had no real understanding of and hope for the future…until I met the man I didn't marry.

What I Did Wrong
- Waited a long time to get any kind of help for my depression and anxiety even though I knew it wasn't normal and that it wasn't just going to go away on its own, no matter how much I wanted it to.
- Didn't take the time to seek out the right kind of help when I did finally go looking for treatment.
- Took the doctor's advice of not looking up symptoms and possible side effects until well after I took the medication – you should *always* know what kinds of side effects a new medication can cause.
- Didn't involve myself in my daughter's life enough to see the issues she was really facing, or enough to let her feel safe talking to me, so I could only watch her get worse and worse over time.

- Was so selfish that I didn't realize the damage I was doing to other people's feelings.
- Drove away most of my friends by the poor choices I made, and didn't even try to get them back.

What To Look For
- Not seeking help, even when you know things aren't right either mentally, physically, or both.
- Blindly taking advice without making sure the advice is really right for you.
- Looking for instant help, instead of the right help for what you're facing.
- Not realizing that the way you feel has to be pushed aside in order to care for those who can't care for themselves, like your children. They should be able to come to you with what they're facing, always.
- Losing friends and family members because they can't handle the 'poor me' stereotype that you've created and refuse to shake off.
- Not noticing how much you're hurting others and/or not being sensitive to their needs and feelings.

What The Therapist Says

Few people ever realize how important a good sense of self-worth is in our lives. In a world where the main emphasis appears to be on external things - the right marriage, job, car, house, etc. - we are indoctrinated with the idea that our worth comes from what we have and what others think of us. The possibility that there might be something about us that is intrinsically worthwhile, even during times when we behave badly, is a foreign concept to most of us. Ironically, on an intellectual level even the very founders of this country acknowledged a certain degree of unconditional self-acceptance when they stated that we were endowed with certain "inalienable rights." Yet emotionally we make our self-worth dependent on how we act and what we achieve.

It is easy to see then how we are drawn to seek external solutions when we feel empty or worthless inside. These solutions may be medication, working harder, an addictive behavior, anything that may serve to distract us from our internal emptiness and fill that void. Especially when low self-esteem leads to severe depression, anxiety, or other mood disorders this need for a quick fix becomes extremely powerful. And that is understandable. As stated before, we do not want to be in pain and will try to escape it as quickly as possible. In the case of the mental conditions mentioned before, certain kinds of medication may not only be appropriate but actually essential at one point or another. Where many a person with low self-worth and depression makes his mistake is by assuming that taking a pill is all that is required to solve his problems.

Medication can help stabilize an individual's depressive moods or anxiety symptoms. It may even ease the pain of low self-esteem to bearable levels. What it cannot do is actually undo the subconscious beliefs that contributed to both the mood disorders and the addictive behaviors in the first place. Medication is intended to ease emotional distress to a point where the sufferer will become stable enough to then engage in the therapy and self-improvement that can address all the subconscious attitudes that cause him or her distress. Sadly, many do not engage in that second, important step of betterment and choose instead to remain dependent on the medication as their sole means of support – another external source of support. In some cases people may suffer from true physical issues that add to their anxiety and mood concerns. In such cases, like schizophrenia, obsessive-compulsive disorders, or bipolar disorders, medication may be required indefinitely. But even in these cases medication alone will not be sufficient to help the sufferer move toward a state of healthier self-image.

So what can a person who is suffering from codependence caused by an innate idea of low self-worth do to get better? Seeking help from a professional therapist would be one avenue, particularly as an outside observer may be able to better discern the addictive patterns in the relationship addict's life and relate them to the past experiences that caused low self-esteem. But even without therapy there are a number of sources and tools for self-improvement out there that have been proven to be extremely effective. Some of the most effective ones look so simple or even silly on the surface that many people do not engage in them. It is another false assumption harbored by our society that only things that are complicated are effective in dealing with serious problems.

Good examples of the simplest of these techniques are self-affirmations. In their most basic form all self-affirmations are is telling ourselves positive things. Sounds simple, and a bit silly at first glance, doesn't it? After all, if we think of someone standing in front of their bathroom mirror talking to their own reflection, saying something nice to themselves, the usual emotional response we get is to think the person in question must be a pathetic loser. Maybe that person is suffering from schizophrenia? The possibility that the activity in question may be the execution of a purposeful and carefully designed self-improvement technique is probably one of the last to enter our minds. Again, this is a reflection of the values and expectations our culture has indoctrinated us with rather than a reflection of truth. In order for us to gain the benefit of many self-help methods that can improve our self-worth we may be forced to ignore those immediate judgments and devaluations. That can be difficult. The last thing people with low self-esteem want to do is feel even more pathetic. One way to overcome this aversion to using self-affirmation, the practice of saying nice things to our own self, is to understand the scientific backing behind it.

A few chapters ago I first pointed out the way our subconscious mind learns, gathers experience, and then draws its conclusions from those experiences. Those conclusions shape the innermost attitudes and beliefs we hold about ourselves and the world. Remember that the subconscious does that through experience alone, experience that has to have some sort of physical or emotional response to it in order to make an impression on our subconscious. Rational thought or simply trying to mentally convince ourselves of something rarely, if ever, makes one bit of difference to those deeply ingrained patterns of belief. This simple fact serves as an explanation of why it is so difficult to change codependent attitudes and addictive behaviors simply by understanding where they come from and how irrational they are. We need a physical way to get new experiences, experiences that the subconscious mind will believe and listen to, in order for it to accept new ideas about our self-worth.

This is where self-affirmations come in. Try to imagine the same scenario I mentioned above from the point of view of our subconscious mind. A person is standing in front of the bathroom mirror saying nice things to him or herself. The body is actively seeing the reflection, meaning the person these compliments are being addressed to. That would be one physical input the subconscious gets. Our mouths experience us saying good things about ourselves. Now the subconscious mind does not care about whether we believe what we say in this moment. It only records the data presented to it and then draws its own conclusions later. It experiences us saying something nice to our own self. In its own association the following conclusions will be drawn: (1) I usually only say things I mean or that are true, and (2) If I say nice things about myself, they might be true. Again, whether we believe in what we say at the point in time we say it does not matter. What matters is that we supply our memory with this experience, so it can be stored and, if stored enough times, then be used to draw new conclusions about our own worth.

Two factors are very important in this process. The first one being the aforementioned notion that we do not need to actually believe what we say. The first time people who try this technique say things like, "you are great just the way you are" or "you are a good and worthwhile person," they do not believe a single word they are saying. But that does not matter at all. The second factor is repetition. Just as our previous sense of self-acceptance was formed through experiences we had over and over again, we need to repeat the retraining steps many times as well, so that our subconscious can begin to change its views. Brushing and flossing your teeth are a good example. We do not expect to do that once in our lifetime and then assume we will have clean teeth for the rest of our lives. It is the same way with affirmations. They have to become a habit to be effective.

Making sure to engage in self-affirmations each morning is a good start. And there are alternative means of doing that, means that may feel less silly than saying them out loud in front of the mirror. Another way would be to write a few affirmations we would like to believe and feel on a card we then read repeatedly every morning, just as we would brush our teeth every morning. The process of reading is another experience to the subconscious mind. It is important, though, to engage in the behavior on a regular basis. In a way, it can serve as a kind of "mental floss." Over time the habit will become more and more automatic and the subconscious mind will begin to internalize these new messages. I use a variation of this technique myself and it has done wonders for my life. Many of the other techniques I will describe in later chapters all have the aspect of repetitious and continuous use in common. That is one concession a codependency sufferer may have to make and understand. In order to maintain a healthy sense of inner worth, we have to do just that: *maintain it*. It is not a one-shot fix. Just as old attitudes of low self-esteem get reinforced every day by old codependent and addictive behaviors, the new improved self-esteem needs to be reiterated over and over again. Thankfully, after a while, those new processes also become second nature.

Chapter 9: I Almost Did it Again – How the Pattern was Broken

In the summer of 2006 I joined an anxiety message board on the Internet in the hope of talking to others 'like me.' It was my way of vaguely trying to help myself, but it was also my new way of seeking validation from others. At that time, I still thought anxiety and depression were my only problems. Despite everything I'd been through, I refused to acknowledge that I had a problem with relationships where men and marriages were concerned, and that I had a problem with my family relationships as well. It was one thing not to have a name for the problem, but it was another thing entirely not to accept that it was there at all. I wasn't willing to admit there was another flaw in me, or that I needed help. I was too stubborn. I was already carrying the shame of the failed relationships and the knowledge that I was blaming them on others. I was already carrying the anxiety, depression, and lack of self-esteem. I was already carrying my feeling that I could never be good enough for my parents – especially not now. I was already carrying the belief that God didn't love me anymore. I refused to pour anything else into my bowl of guilt and misery. Fortunately for me, I was also still carrying that little spark that was glowing deep down inside, and the nagging thought that it was time for a change.

Originally I wasn't going to bother to join the anxiety board, since I could read everyone else's comments without signing up, but I had another one of those 'gut feelings' and this time it was way too strong to ignore, so I rationalized the idea that it might be a good choice and was cheaper than therapy. I couldn't afford to see anyone about my anxiety, and I wouldn't have done it anyway. I wasn't raised to do that sort of thing, and at the time I thought only weak people went to therapy. It's amazing how our views change. The idea of getting 'therapy' anonymously through the anxiety board seemed like it made a lot of sense. By using that as a logical argument I could feel like I *thought* about the decision and made it rationally instead of going by a 'feeling.' I had been raised to think about things, and even though the idea of 'following your heart' was intriguing to me, I still couldn't break the old habit of rationalization. If it didn't make logical sense (at least to me through whatever justification I could find) then I wasn't going to do it. Period. So I joined the message board and made a few posts, but then my anxiety just melted away. I thought it was gone...back into remission. How wonderful! Maybe all I'd needed was that willingness to join a help group. That had been the magic cure I was looking for, and I hadn't even needed to work for it. Perfect.

I felt absolutely great for about four days, and because of that I went and unsubscribed from the anxiety board. I figured there was no reason for staying on it if I didn't have anxiety any more. I didn't need any more help. Those four days were wonderful...I almost felt like I was going to have a great future after all; that there was hope for me yet. On the morning of the fifth day I was slammed with a huge panic attack, right out of the blue, just to let me know I shouldn't be getting ahead of myself, I guess. I don't know what caused it or where it came from but it was definitely there, and it wasn't going away. For three days I fought with it. I tried to ignore it, I tried to be angry at it, I tried anything I could think of to make it go away again, but nothing worked. I couldn't sleep well, and I ate very little. Misery was starting to settle in again, and I didn't want to let it. At the same time my brain kept nagging me about the anxiety board. I wasn't interested.

I told myself I didn't need that. I wasn't sick. I thought if I believed it long enough it would be true...but the problem was that I didn't *really* believe it. Finally I found myself re-joining the board late one night when I couldn't sleep and couldn't keep my mind on my work. I had been anxious for three days straight...not always in a panic attack, but always in a heightened state of anxiety...and always with the message board on my mind, running around and around in my head and not giving me a moment's peace. It was wearing me down in a big way. Finally I decided to accept that there might be a point to this. Maybe there was more to this than met the eye, or that made sense logically. Maybe there was a 'message' to or on the message board. Maybe God was trying to tell me something after all...was it possible He still cared about what happened to me? So I signed back up. The way things were going, I felt like I didn't have a lot of choice.

Signing up again didn't take my anxiety away but it did give me a sense of relief, and a feeling that at least I had people to talk to who understood what I was going through. I didn't know anyone else with anxiety who I could talk to in person, and meeting others – even through the Internet – made me feel more human and more normal. Of course, I still wouldn't acknowledge what my *real* issues were and try to deal with them. Anxiety and depression were far from my only problems…and my most serious problem was about to rear its ugly head again, in a way that would forever alter the course of my life. I met a man.

His name was Klaus, and he was a moderator on the board. He was always commenting on people's posts with a kind word and a smiley face icon, and it seemed like he was knowledgeable and generally good-hearted. In the few days I had been off the board someone else had started a thread about 'all of us panic people' meeting up with one another. Most people laughed at that. Travel outside of our individual comfort zones? Yeah, right. Sure. Some of them were too afraid to even leave their own homes or drive on the freeway. Many of them would never consider a trip beyond the borders of their town. How amusing, they all thought, when it was suggested. Klaus, however, said that he would love to meet other sufferers. I read the post. When I signed back up on the board I knew I *had* to answer it. I don't even know why. I just did. I would have to say that post was the single most significant reason that caused me to sign up again. The anxiety I was continuing to experience was a close second, though. Klaus lived 500 miles away from me and I knew virtually nothing about him, but something about him struck me and I couldn't get him out of my head. Still I found myself wondering: would he come visit?

I responded to the post and we talked on the thread, back and forth, for a little while. From there we sent private emails through the board, and then we exchanged personal email addresses so we could talk more frequently and see if we had anything in common. We did have a few things…we were both Christians, we both drove the same style of car and liked some of the same music, food, and television shows. We both liked to laugh, but hadn't had much to laugh about lately. He gave me his phone number and the idea of calling him made me incredibly nervous, but I did it anyway. It was another exciting adventure and it was OK, I told myself, because he had anxiety, too. That would make it better this time. The first time I called him we both said hello, and then there was silence. "Well, that's all I've got," I finally said, and we both started laughing and the ice was broken. We ended up talking for two hours, with me closing my eyes often and just listening to his voice – he had the cutest accent I'd ever heard! Faint and not overdone, but enough you could place the fact he wasn't originally from the United States. Born and raised in Europe, he had moved with his family after high school to go to college here in the U.S.

Since that first phone conversation went so well we continued our emails, and Klaus started calling me almost every day, just to chat. He told me stories from his childhood and talked about the anxiety problems he struggled with. I told him stories about my life, too, but I kept some things back. There was no way I was going to tell this great new guy I'd been divorced five times. He'd never been married…never even had a girlfriend…because of the anxiety, and I was sure he would run screaming if he knew about my past. I didn't see any reason why he ever had to know about any of it. Even if we really fell for each other, I wasn't looking to get married again. I could handle just having a boyfriend. That would be enough, and I'd never have to disclose my past information. He knew about some of it – my daughter's father, for example, and my last marriage, because I told him about the awful things Jack had done while we were together. But being twice-divorced in your mid-thirties is a lot different from being five-times-divorced in your mid-thirties. Better to play my cards close to the chest and just see what happened.

Klaus, from what I could tell over the phone and through email, was a truly nice person. He was also a very funny, very caring, and very joyous person despite his anxiety disorder. We started up a friendship through our phone contact, and then we met in person. I didn't know what to think about meeting him. I was tremendously excited about it but also terribly nervous, and I wasn't sure how well I really knew him. We'd only been talking on the phone and via email for a couple of weeks when he made the 500 mile drive to come to my town.

I met him at the hotel where he was staying. I didn't want him coming to my house and being around my daughter without getting to know him in person for a little while. I wasn't going to risk her safety. I was also concerned that he might be interested in sponging off me financially. He knew what I did for a living and that I had my own house and a nice vehicle. At thirty he was still living with his parents, driving one of their cars, and had no job. I thought he was probably just a polite and well-mannered bum. Turned out he was wealthy and didn't have to work, but I didn't find that out until later.

In person, I liked him right away. He was so friendly and personable...but I didn't feel that spark I had hoped for. I just thought he was nice. We spent a couple of hours together, and then I let him come to my house and meet my daughter. We all had a good time together, just laughing and watching TV and joking around. After he left that night I mentioned to Karyn that I liked Klaus, but I didn't *like* Klaus. I thought it would be a 'friends only' kind of relationship. She got very upset and started crying, almost begging me to give him a chance. This was so unlike her! Normally she shied away from men because of her past stepfathers and the problems my being with them had brought into our lives. She also had a lot of anger at her father, since he wasn't around much. With Klaus, she seemed convinced he mattered to our lives in some way. He was important. She told me many months later, as we sat talking about how our lives had changed, that she just felt as though he would be very significant to our lives, and we mustn't ignore that – it was why she had cried that night, because she didn't know how to convey it properly. She didn't think I would understand. She was right. At the time it was all taking place, I wouldn't have understood.

The next day, for her sake, I tried to look at Klaus with new eyes. He *was* pretty cute, in a very boyish sort of way. He seemed to be genuine...he was just himself, whether others liked it or not. He didn't apologize for much. He was always smiling...unless he was panicking...and he was generous to a fault. Maybe I did like him after all...or maybe I could learn to. He seemed to like me, too, but he was awkward and shy about it. Three days into his visit, while we were sitting on the couch watching TV, I reached over and took his hand. He stared at me, wide-eyed and startled, and then looked down at our clasped hands, resting on my leg.

"I've never held hands with a girl before," he said softly, and then his eyes sought my face again, showing me both his interest and his fright.

I didn't know what to do with this man I was rapidly becoming very interested in. If he'd never held hands before he'd probably never kissed a girl, either, which meant that he'd never...oh dear. I was suddenly *very* uncomfortable. I didn't even mean to think that thought, but there it was. I shoved it to the back of my mind, smiled at him, and we went back to watching TV.

He stayed for five days, and it was difficult for me to let him go. I'd fallen for him hard in the few days he'd been in my life, but he had to get back to where he lived. He had pets to take care of, and his parents were about to head out on yet another trip in just a couple of weeks. He needed to go home, but it was clear he wanted to stay as well. Saying goodbye was difficult for both of us, and we dragged it out as much as we could. Right before he left we walked down by the water near his hotel and he picked up a seashell and handed it to me, requesting that I take it home for Karyn. He thought she'd like it. I agreed. He held it up to the light and pronounced it empty. After he drove away I went home and gave her the shell. She put it on her desk. Fifteen minutes later she came out and poked her head around the corner of the living room, her eyes huge. I looked up from my spot on the couch and when my gaze met hers I had a moment of perfect clarity.

"It's walking across your desk isn't it?" I asked.

She nodded, still big-eyed, and we both started laughing. A hermit crab had made its home in that shell, Klaus hadn't noticed it, and Mr. Crab wasn't happy on a big expanse of wood. Still laughing, we carried the tiny creature back down to the water and turned him loose to go on and do whatever it is that hermit crabs do.

I talked to Klaus every day on the phone, and we emailed as well. I liked him a great deal, but I also liked his money. I'd be lying if I said otherwise. I'd never been wealthy, and didn't expect to ever be. My self-esteem wasn't high enough to let me think I was good enough for that. The writing I was doing had become just another job to me, and I no longer found much enjoyment in it. I was surviving financially, but I couldn't seem to get ahead. Most of my life I'd lived payday to payday, sometimes with literally as little as twenty dollars in the bank to get me through until I got paid again. I had a bit more than that by the time I met Klaus, but not much. The idea that a rich man would think I was worthy of a second look was a thought I hadn't really entertained before, but I was thinking about it then.

I felt very lucky, but I also thought about all the nice things I would like to have. Could I get those things from him? Could I stop working? Could I live a life of luxury? It wasn't so much greed…I didn't want fur coats and big diamond rings…as it was just a desire not to have to struggle. I was tired of fighting to pay my bills, tired of worrying about getting sick because I had no health insurance, and tired of not being able to give Karyn much of anything. I wasn't broke, but just getting by was about all I was able to do. Maybe Klaus could change all that, and if we were happy together there would be no harm in being with him. It wasn't *just* for the money, after all.

While we were apart, Klaus took a trip to his native country for a month. He still called me, but only once each day because of the time difference. He would call just before he went to bed, which would be around midday for me. I got to hear about his day and he got to hear about mine. It wasn't long before we were saying 'I love you' before we hung up the phone. Sometimes he would call my answering machine when he knew I wasn't going to be home and sing to me. It was weird, but it was endearing as well. I couldn't get enough of him. He taught me a few foreign words, most of which I promptly forgot, and I learned about some of the societal differences in the way he grew up and the way I grew up. Most of it was fascinating. I also learned he had an obsession with sci-fi, specifically Star Wars, but I could look beyond that. The most important thing was that we were happy. My mother liked him and so did Karyn. My father said very little. He was probably thinking 'here we go again,' and he would have been right – sort of.

There was a problem, though. Klaus still didn't know about my multiple marriages, and it was nagging at me. I had guilt. I knew it wasn't fair to him, and I felt like I was living a lie. I had to tell him the whole truth but I didn't know how – and I was terrified he would walk away, either because he felt like I had lied to him or because he couldn't imagine dating someone who went through husbands at such an alarming rate. What if he left me? I wasn't sure I could bear that…I really, really thought I'd found my chance at happiness by meeting him. I had, but it wasn't going to turn out the way I thought it would. Have you ever wanted something so much and you get something else and realize it's even better? It came to me through Klaus, but first I had to go through the growing pains of the relationship. The patterns I followed weren't that easily changed or broken. For once in my life where a relationship was concerned, I did the right thing – I told Klaus the complete truth…but I have to admit he gave me an easy opening to discuss the issue, and some accidental guilt to go along with it before I was persuaded to come clean.

While he was still on his trip he sent me an email. He had a confession to make, he said, and he needed to get it off his chest. Uh-oh. I wasn't sure what to expect, but it turned out not to be that horrible. It was something I could live with, didn't involve anything illegal, had nothing to do with another woman, and wasn't something I felt I had a huge problem with. It was in the past. Since he was confessing, I knew it was now or never for me to be honest with him. If I didn't do it now and he ever found out…who knew what might happen then? He'd been honest with me, and if I didn't return the favor I feared the guilt would eventually consume me. So I replied to his email and told him it was OK and that I understood, and then I told him the truth about my failed marriages – well, *my* truth, which probably wasn't the same as my ex-husbands' truths. Still, I was honest about the number of divorces I'd racked up, and I admitted how scared I was that he would never speak to me again, but I could understand it if that was what he needed to do. And then I cried. Hard. For a long time…well into the night. I couldn't sleep, and when I had exhausted all my tears I dozed fitfully, wishing I had never sent that message.

I looked at the clock at about 2:55 a.m., and I had another one of those weird, intuitive thoughts that seem to come from nowhere. This one said the phone was going to ring, and two minutes later it did. It was Klaus, saying it was OK and he loved me and there was *no chance* he would leave me over something like this. He knew it was the middle of the night where I was but he figured I wouldn't be sleeping well and he didn't want me to worry any more. It wasn't even a big deal to him. He didn't care! All that angst and worry and all those tears and *he didn't even care!* I was overjoyed; so happy I started crying again, for a totally different reason this time. We laughed and cried on the phone for a few minutes, and he promised to call me at a saner hour, and we said our goodbyes. I was finally able to get to sleep and Karyn, who'd been awakened by the ringing phone – on a school night – wasn't even upset. She knew how worried I'd been in sending that email, and she felt only relief that things worked out the way they did. It was a huge weight lifted off my shoulders. That doesn't mean I wasn't still ashamed of my past, but only that I was glad I no longer had to lie to Klaus about it.

When Klaus got back from his trip he came to see me again, with the idea of finding a place to live near me. Instead of getting a hotel while he looked for a rental, I just let him stay at my house. The first night he lied next to me, shaking, too scared to do anything but panic. Finally he reached one hand out, hooked his pinky finger through mine, and we fell asleep that way. It was totally innocent and very loving, and I felt no pressure for rapid physical involvement, which was great. It wasn't something I was used to and it made me even more certain I was doing the right thing by spending my time with Klaus and by being honest with him. In a few days Klaus found a rental house about ten minutes from me and then went home to get his things, showing up a week later with a truck full of stuff and his father. I was overjoyed to meet his dad…he was a nice man and seemed genuinely pleased his son had found someone who made him happy. He was also a good-looking man for his age, and the accent helped. I was a sucker for that accent. Klaus and his rich, foreign family all seemed so exotic. He stayed for a couple of days and we all enjoyed our time together. Klaus moved his things into the rental and set up a nice little home for himself – and didn't live in it.

We couldn't seem to be able to be apart. He spent his days and nights with me, and our relationship was comfortable and happy. I worked less and it was cutting into my finances, a concept which was completely alien to him. After only a few short months of this I woke him from a nap one afternoon and he pulled me down on the bed with him and looked at me for a long moment.

"I wonder what our wedding will be like?" he asked, completely out of the blue.

I had no clue he even *wanted* to marry me. For once, I was reasonably content to have a boyfriend. He was helping with the housework and we were spending time with Karyn, who was slowly starting to come out of her shell. She and Klaus both shared a passion for painting, and that gave them some common ground on which to bond. I've never been an artist, so it was something that was just for the two of them. They looked at each other's work, compared notes, collaborated, and seemed to be enjoying themselves. Unlike with some of the men I'd been with in the past, I never worried about Klaus having any sort of romantic ideas about Karyn. Even though she already looked like a woman, he truly understood that looks could be deceiving. She was still a child.

Everything was good just the way it was, so what in the world was he doing mentioning marriage? I had my brain set on 'boyfriend,' but we were so happy together! Why shouldn't we get married? It made sense, since we were already living in the same house and it seemed to be working well. His pets liked my pets, and Karyn seemed happier, as well. He had a good personality and was a caring person…and there was the money, of course. While I wouldn't have married him just to have the money, it was certainly not to be discounted. It was the proverbial icing on the cake. There was one issue. His parents. It's not that I didn't like them, it's just that they seemed not to like *me*. Or rather, they seemed not to *trust* me. I guess I couldn't blame them. They didn't know about the multiple marriages but they did know I was divorced, and since I wasn't rich I guess they assumed I was a gold digger. Or it might not have even been anything personal or have anything to do with me. Perhaps they just didn't trust anyone where money was concerned, and

I'm sure they were interested in protecting Klaus...but when he had to call them and ask whether they thought the money he was going to spend on my engagement ring (a very modest amount) was too much I started to wonder just how much control they had over his life – and how much they would have over mine. Then came the prenup.

When they started hounding Klaus to make a prenuptial agreement, I balked. No. I wasn't signing it. Why should I? Klaus and I were adults. I didn't want a prenup and neither did he, so we shouldn't have one, right? Right. Except for his parents. He was concerned about pleasing them, and he often did what they wanted or agreed to their demands to keep the peace or to feel accepted and loved, just like I was always doing with my parents. I never really realized how incredibly annoying it was until I had to deal with someone else who was involved in it. It caused us to have our first big fight, which continued – on and off – for several days. Finally his parents won – kind of. We did create a prenuptial agreement, but we wrote it ourselves in plain language and in terms we were both happy with, and we carried it down to a local notary and signed it. Klaus' dad didn't even ask to see it! It was enough for him to know we had done it, apparently. Why didn't we just *say* we had done it? I don't know. The whole thing was kind of surreal, really. But I had my ring and we combined our funds and our furniture and everything, and we started planning the wedding.

When we set a date we had about six months to get ready, which we thought would be no problem. After all, I'd done this before. He bought his tuxedo, I bought a dress, and we went about getting all the other little details ready. One thing we wanted was butterflies. We saw them everywhere we went, and once we even drove through a big cloud of them, not harming a single one. It was strange. Klaus claimed to be big into meditation, energy healing, spirituality, and things like that, and he took the butterflies as a sign. After they continued to appear everywhere I looked, I started to concede that he might be right. I still wasn't completely sure how I felt about that. To me any of that other alternative spirituality stuff was almost like Voodoo or something. With my sheltered youth and closed-in understanding of the world I thought it was anti-Christian. I hadn't yet expanded my mind to the fact there were other possibilities for religious opinion than what I'd been taught. I tried not to think too much about it because I was about to marry this man, and I didn't want something screwing that up. I had a chance at a real, secure future for Karyn and me, and blowing that would be stupid. Klaus and I finally found a place that had a lot of butterflies around virtually all the time, and it was beautiful and right near the water. It seemed like it would be a great place for a wedding, and because it was in a public park it was free for us to use it.

Klaus was sometimes a penny pincher, almost to the point of being stingy. I didn't expect him to spend hundreds of thousands on our wedding, but he seemed to want to do everything as cheaply as possible. I had virtually no say in the matter but his parents definitely did, and I started wondering about that, as well. It crossed my mind that maybe he didn't think we were as equal as I'd hoped. It was becoming more and more clear that it was still very much *his* money, and not ours. I understood that, and yet I didn't. After all, it was money he brought to the marriage…but if we were really going to share our lives, we should share everything. I didn't restrict where he went in the house because my name was on the deed, did I? It wasn't even about how much he was spending – or not spending – it was about control. He had too much of it and I didn't have enough when it came to the finances, and that caused friction. The thought of not marrying him didn't even cross my mind, though; not at that point. I was still too focused on the fact we could share our panic attacks with one another and really *understand* what it was like. That was very important to me, and to him as well. So I overlooked the control issue, and the mood swings, and the way he always wanted to talk about what he was going through but not so much about what I needed to address.

I tried to keep my concerns to myself, because I was getting a lot of the things I wanted. It seemed like a fair trade. I have to admit my motives weren't entirely pure. There was the money of course, and the security for Karyn with paying for college and all, and there was also the vasectomy. I'd been saying for years I wanted to meet a great guy with a vasectomy so I didn't have to worry about getting pregnant again. As it turned out, Klaus didn't want to pass anxiety on to a new generation and had made a personal decision years earlier not to have children of his own. He was also concerned because both of his parents and his siblings had some other emotional problems and issues, with depression and bipolar disorder running strongly through his family tree. He *wanted* to go and have the procedure done, and of course I was all for it. Things were working out perfectly for me from a logistical standpoint. I thought I could gain control of him from his parents eventually and that would give me more financial control over our situation as well. Then I wouldn't be so much at his mercy when it came to what we as a couple could spend on things…and maybe I could stop working, too. Right then, he wouldn't allow it – he wasn't going to pay my way. I was still going to go through with the marriage even though my feathers were a little ruffled, for Karyn's financial security and because I still believed I could adjust the future to get all of what I wanted in the end. If it weren't for the vasectomy, though, my life probably wouldn't have changed like it did.

When he went for his pre-op appointment I went with him, and on the way back he totally altered the course of my life. With a song. He didn't even mean to, and at the time I didn't realize how deeply it was going to affect me. I know how silly that must sound, of course I do, but everyone has something that resonates with them. Something that makes them happy no matter what. Something that makes them see things differently. They just have to find what that 'something' is. For me, that something is music. I've always liked music, all different types and styles, everything from classical operas to death metal to country to rap, but I didn't realize the depth of enjoyment that music could actually give me. I didn't realize how important it could be. I wasn't aware of the power that it had. But I was about to be enlightened. Klaus and I were driving along, heading home from his doctor's appointment, when he asked if he could play one of those mix CDs that have all kinds of different songs from different artists on them. I shrugged. I was listening to something I liked at that moment and I didn't really want to change that, but I didn't want to be rude, either. My biggest concern was that the CD was a German one, and I expected to get stuck with a lot of beer drinking 'oompah' music if I let him play it. This was different, though. It was a pretty good song, with the exception of the fact I had absolutely no idea what the words were. I couldn't tell you what it was now, though. I don't remember what it sounded like or who sang it. It wasn't important to me.

When it was over the next song came on and Klaus went to take the CD out.

"You don't want to hear that one," he said. "It's hip-hop."

I grabbed his hand and moved it away from the CD player. "I like hip-hop. Leave it be."

The song played through, and I made him play it again. And once more. I think I understood maybe three or four words of it, and whoever was singing was moving at what I thought was a highly impressive rate of speed. Have you ever heard someone say they heard a particular piece of music and because of it they were never the same? It's usually some aria or a significant classical piece. Something dramatic and haunting. For me, it's German hip-hop. I could try to explain why, but since I don't understand it myself it would be a pretty short explanation. Like I said, everyone has something that resonates with them, and that style of music in that particular language was it for me. It made me happy – joyous, actually – and I started to write more again, just for pleasure.

Karyn had fallen in love with the music, too, and encouraged me to continue listening to it and to continue writing and dreaming. Those were things I hadn't done for a long time. Most of my dreams had died in the middle of anxiety, depression, and bad marriages, and I only wrote what I had to so I could pay the bills. I hadn't written what *I* wanted to write, just for sheer pleasure, in a very long time. Suddenly writing was becoming fun again, and that renewed interest actually helped in my work. I started setting better deadlines for myself and getting through my work for the clients I had at the time more quickly so I could turn in my assignments and go back to working on the things I wanted to write. Everything about the situation made me smile – except, for some reason, Klaus.

I was still basically happy with him and our relationship but there were little aggravations I was becoming more aware of; things I hadn't seen before. He could be childish, and arrogant, and self-centered. I suppose it was mostly the way he was raised. When you come from wealth and privilege you often do things far differently from the rest of the world. It was nothing for him to jet off to somewhere just because, or to buy something he wanted, only to throw it away a month later because it broke. Money meant nothing to him when he was spending it on his own pursuits, but getting any of it from him for anything else was like pulling teeth. And that wasn't our only problem. It might have been the most obvious and concrete one, but there were others that were hanging around, too, lurking there waiting to sabotage what I'd originally thought was a good thing.

I really did care for Klaus despite the annoying things I was starting to notice, but about two months before our wedding date it all changed, seemingly in the blink of an eye. Klaus started acting much more panicky and I started having a lot of problems, too, just when I'd begun to feel better overall. I realized I was thinking too much about money and travel, and he didn't seem to be thinking at all…only worrying and getting more and more stressed out over everything. A lot of questions ran around my brain in the days that followed as his mood swings and panic attacks became more severe. I wanted to be with him, but was it for the wrong reasons? And why was he with me? Did he really *love* me? Was he really *in love* with me? Or was it only that I was his first in everything and he felt like that counted for something? Maybe he just didn't want to be alone? I had a million questions going through my head and no good answers, so I did what I'd found always helped me since the day I discovered it. I turned on 'my' music and it made me happy and peaceful and joyous. How strange – and how wonderful – that something so obscure would become so important in my life. If it wasn't for Klaus I would have no idea that this music existed. I owed him. But did I owe him *marriage*? Did he even still *want* marriage?

I talked him into going to see a doctor. Maybe the anxiety medication he was taking wasn't working well anymore? After taking a careful history, his doctor diagnosed him as bipolar – not a huge surprise, since it was in his family – and gave him a new medication to try. He'd probably had the disorder all along and had been wrongly diagnosed in the past as having only anxiety. Upon getting this diagnosis Klaus announced he'd decided we shouldn't live together any more, at least until he straightened his life and his moods out a bit on the new medication, so he took his cats and moved out. Since he still had the rental house and most of his furniture was still in it, at least he had a home to go to. I would've felt horrible if he had to stay in a hotel all alone, but when he left it was a huge weight off my and Karyn's shoulders – and I believe off Klaus' as well. I think that was the point when he and I both knew marriage was no longer really a good option for us. He didn't want to put me through living with him the way he was, and I didn't want to put Karyn through the ups and downs that came with it, but I told him I wouldn't turn my back on him. He couldn't help the fact that he was ill. It wasn't like it was his fault or that he'd asked for it, just like I hadn't asked for my own problems. But I knew when we both realized we didn't miss living together there was more to it than just mental health issues.

Karyn and I had gotten much closer while Klaus was living with us, and I think that mattered to her much more than I'd ever thought it would. Even though we both still panicked sometimes and both still had days where we were depressed or just plain didn't feel right, our quality of life was vastly improved from what it'd been before Klaus had come into our lives. When things started going wrong I didn't fall apart like I would've expected to. I thought for a while we could work it out, and then later I thought it would be all right regardless of whether we could work it out or not. It wasn't the same as the marriages of the past where we fought all the time and accused each other of horrible things – sometimes with very good reason. This was just two people who were struggling to find who they were and what they were supposed to be getting out of their lives, and they'd grown so much while they were together that now they were growing apart. I could see our lives heading off in different directions, and I didn't know how to stop it…or whether I should even try. I was sad, and yet I wasn't.

Ultimately, Klaus made the choice not to marry. He thought we'd all be better off that way, and I respected that decision. We'd already mailed out the invitations, but we talked it out and decided neither one of us really wanted to get married after all, for a lot of reasons. He said it wasn't only my 'obsession' with the music I fell in love with, but there was just something that was causing him to panic over the whole thing, and it went far beyond 'cold feet.' It was a giving up of freedom and lifestyle he wasn't willing or ready to accept. The bipolar disorder was a contributing factor, but it wasn't all of it. I respected his honesty and agreed with his conclusions...I didn't know precisely why it was, but the whole idea of the wedding was just hitting me wrong. I didn't even know how to explain it to him. It wasn't a lack of love, but I did have some concerns over some of his actions, ideas, and opinions. I still felt like he thought he was privileged, and that he believed he was better than me because he'd come from wealth and I had not. I didn't see that ever going away, or him ever truly treating me as an equal. It wasn't his fault – he didn't know how to. I was surprised I didn't feel bad about our decision, but I actually felt as though what we had decided on was the right thing to do.

For some reason I didn't feel rejected, or lost, or not good enough, or anything. I had my enjoyment of writing back, and I had music...which was playing a huge role in helping me get my enjoyment of *life* back. Karyn was laughing more. You could see the change in her mannerisms, her schoolwork, and her attitude in general. She began to take some pride in herself again, and so did I. Things were better than they'd been in a very, very long time, even though I wasn't getting married. I had a real life, with real interests that were just my own, for the first time that I could remember. But Klaus and I had planned to marry, and it was hard to write notes to follow those invitations, saying the wedding was off. How could I explain it? There wasn't any way to do that. It's not like I wanted to tell the world about Klaus' bipolar problems or the issues he'd grappled with, and I knew my family – most of them probably wouldn't have understood my music revelation, and they likely wouldn't even try to. So I wrote notes that just said that, after much discussion, we had reached the conclusion that neither one of us was ready to marry at this point in time, and I sent them out. Not one person responded to say they were glad, sorry, or anything else. I guess they didn't really know what to say. As for me, I was both saddened and overjoyed at the same time, but I'll admit I mourned the loss of the money. Who wouldn't? The security I thought I'd have and be able to give to Karyn had just evaporated.

But it was the first time in my life that *not* getting married had made me happy in any way. It was what I needed…it was like a big bubble just popped. Oh, don't get me wrong, it didn't take away my anxiety and it didn't magically fix everything, but it *did* show me I could be alone and still be a whole person. I didn't need others to make me complete. I wasn't defined by being a 'Mrs.' Apparently Klaus had come into my life for a reason, and now he'd fulfilled his purpose. Karyn was right…he ended up being very important to us. He didn't come to save me, but to show me a way in which I could save myself, which was ultimately much more valuable. If someone else saves you, you need them to continue to do it. If they teach you to save yourself, you can always use what you've learned, no matter what the other person does or if he or she is still in your life.

Klaus and I continued to date for a little while after he moved out but it was somehow awkward, and we turned it into a friendship I still value very highly. It's been surprisingly easy to make that transition. Sometimes we hug a bit longer than we should, but we are *friends*, and that's what we'll stay. I have no desire to go back, and I don't think he does either. I will never forget, though, that he gave me the opportunity to discover that I could be happy on my own. All I needed was some renewed faith in myself and my abilities. All I needed was something besides one specific man that made me feel like life was worth living again – and now I had that. Coupled with my renewed love of writing and Karyn's increased happiness it was enough, both for me and for Karyn. I didn't get married when I had the chance! The devastating pattern by which I had lived my life for so long had been broken. I was finally free from myself.

What I Did Wrong

- Avoided trying to get to the root of the problem and solve it until I was forced to really confront it.

- Tried to ignore that 'inner voice' that I really should have been listening to all along, and focused only on what appeared 'logical' instead.
- Started a new relationship on a lie, by not telling him about the number of past marriages and divorces I'd experienced.
- Didn't insist that we live apart so that we could really get to know one another.
- Entertained the thought of marrying again even though I'd already failed at it five times.
- Didn't take into account that it really is very difficult to marry outside one's social and financial class, and there are always issues that come along with that.
- Still saw my relationship as revolving around who had control of everything.
- Focused too much on money and security and not enough on the love and caring that should have gone into the relationship.

What To Look For
- Dealing with *a* problem you have but not dealing with *the* problem you have.
- Ignoring that 'inner voice' that keeps nagging you and trying to steer you in the right direction.
- Lying in a relationship because you don't feel you can be who you are and still be accepted.
- Focusing on anything other than love for your partner (sex, money, possessions, etc.).
- Not taking enough time to be apart from someone and get to know them before living together and/or marrying.
- Social class, finances, religion, etc. shouldn't matter, but they often do. These things have to be thoroughly addressed to get past them. They don't go away on their own.
- Worrying about control, instead of sharing it.

- Getting involved with someone again, without getting help first, when it's clear that you haven't done well at it in the past.

What The Therapist Says

This chapter shows a lot of things to be possible that many people with codependent concerns, especially at a time when they recognize their own self-defeating patterns but feel they are trapped within them, do not think could ever be possible. First of all, many love and relationship addicts feel terrified about sharing their shame and experiences with others. As frightening as the prospect of facing one's issues may be and as mortifying as disclosing these issues with others may appear, joining peer support groups can prove to be an amazing asset in recovery of almost any kind. Researching what services and self-help groups are available either in one's own community or through Internet resources can yield amazing opportunities. Sometimes simply realizing that one is not alone in one's dilemma and that other people, who seem nice and lovable, share similar stories, can already serve to raise a codependency sufferer's self-worth.

A mention should be made at this point of a resource that has been proven not only extremely helpful to people suffering from relationship addiction and codependence, but is also one of the more widely accessible and long-standing peer support groups dealing with this subject matter. Codependents Anonymous (CoDA) is based on the twelve-step format pioneered by Alcoholics Anonymous (AA) and, like so many similar twelve-step programs, has given aid and relief to sufferers of its specific group focus, in this case codependency, for many years. The success of twelve-step programs is undeniable even though a number of professional therapists choose to ignore this fact. That is understandable because of two factors. The first deals with the twelve-step programs incorporating a high degree of spiritual ideas, which may clash with an individual's or therapist's own beliefs. Secondly, they are sometimes seen as competition by therapists, who then fear the loss of their client base. Personally speaking, I would advocate to any sufferer of relationship addiction and codependence to at least try a twelve-step program that focuses on whatever issues ail him or her. No resource should be dismissed out of hand or be ignored by a therapist when giving clients treatment options.

The second point in this chapter that represents an assumed impossibility on the part of many codependent individuals is not only breaking the old addictive behavior patterns, but that this break in behavior might actually not be painful, or at least less painful than first feared. In most cases the subconscious mind of an individual dealing with relationship addiction does not only hold the belief that in order to feel good a relationship is essential, but it also feels that any loss of such a relationship will automatically lead to increased and maybe unbearable pain. What is interesting to note is that, again, past experience is automatically used by the subconscious to assume future events and outcomes. As the recovery process begins, events such as described in this chapter, the sharing of one's shame and the dissolution of a relationship without the descent into horrible pain, disprove the attitudes of our internalized beliefs that things always turn out the way we fear. Allowing the possibility to enter our minds that despite what we innately fear events may actually not turn out as badly as imagined is a huge step forward. We do not have to believe in such an outcome. Just entertaining the remote possibility can make a huge difference.

At this point I would like to caution any person who is recovering from codependence and relationship addiction not to assume that one way of having a potentially healthy relationship is to seek out a potential mate who is in the same position. While it is true that an understanding of and shared commitment in overcoming codependent attitudes is a great boon for partners, they should not be a desired starting point for recovery. The reason being is that, especially early in the process, the danger of shifting one's focus to the partner rather than one's own internal healing is very great. We have to remember that a hallmark of the internal attitudes that fuel relationship addiction, low self-worth, and codependence is to seek an external source for validation. To engage in a relationship at such an early stage can easily shift the sufferer's focus to the partner to such a degree that recovery becomes short-circuited.

Another important concept that can be useful in recovery from codependence and related addictive behaviors is the use of any kind of artistic expression. Many times people with low self-worth not only minimize their own value but also the worth of their own emotions. That can manifest itself in a number of ways. While in an addictive relationship the addict might try to minimize his or her sadness over the partner's bad behaviors because the addict does not want to risk jeopardizing the partnership. The way the sufferer does that can occur in various ways. Some simply try to suppress what they feel. Others turn anger and frustration caused by the partner against themselves, shifting the blame to an imagined fault of theirs. In either case the result is that the codependent person devalues his or her emotions. Since emotional responses do not disappear when we suppress them they often get channeled into different forms, causing or aggravating depression, anxiety, and even physical ailments such as fibromyalgia, IBS, or autoimmune disorders. Artistic expression of any kind can be a very powerful tool that allows the relationship addict to reconnect with those denied feelings.

In the case described in this chapter music was the medium, which gave the codependent individual a means to feel and express her own emotions. Music, poetry, and works of art can be great mirrors, in which we can face those deep feelings within us that we would otherwise try so hard to ignore and suppress. Beyond the use of such media to experience these emotions, art can also be functional in expressing them when we actively engage in it. This can range from simply singing along with a tune that echoes what we feel inside to actively creating a work of art that expresses our innermost hopes, dreams, and pains. In this manner the addict can begin to break the pattern of disregarding his or her own feelings and, rather than trying to suppress them, express them in a healthier form. Writing, drawing, pottery, carving, painting, even things like gardening and cooking can serve as creative outlets to release negative emotions and grow positive experiences.

As such, a creative outlet is not only a personal fancy but represents an important tool for recovering a healthier sense of self-acceptance. Many people, through subconscious attitudes, see artistic expression as a childish pastime. In reality it is a most deeply rooted and needed release mechanism for pain and longing that has been part of the human experience ever since we discovered how to dab a cave wall with ochre paints. I would encourage anyone on the path of personal recovery to find one or more creative outlets for themselves. They are invaluable tools for establishing a healthier rapport with one's own emotions. Not only that, by taking the time to engage in this use of art we send an important message to our subconscious mind. We recognize the importance of this emotional outlet, which puts a sense of importance on our own emotional wellbeing. Plus, by engaging in such activities we tell our subconscious that our own feelings are not only important, but that we have enough intrinsic worth in our own self to warrant the use of these creative outlets. The benefit is twofold. We get emotional release and we learn that we are worth taking care of our own needs.

At this point a short caution should be made. While art, in all its forms, can serve as a great outlet for our feelings, it does represent an external means of doing so. As with anything that gives us a sense of relief from our pains and a measure of comfort, one has to take care not to turn this new source of external fulfillment into an addiction in itself. Examples of such excesses can be seen in fanatic idol worship of artists, artists disregarding other personal, sometimes vital needs for the sake of engaging in art, or the use of writing to create a fantasy world to use as an escape from reality. Especially with the large popularity of video games and online role-playing venues, we have been graced with ever-growing opportunities of escaping our reality and potentially our own self. Making sure that we do not abandon our real self for the sake of an "artistic ideal" or "fantasy persona" is very important. Taking this route is a less obvious means of seeking external validation that, after a while, negates our self-worth in the here and now again.

Chapter 10: Relationship Patterns and Spiritual Growth

It wasn't until Klaus seriously started on his own spiritual journey after we ended our romance and settled into our friendship that I felt compelled to start on my own. I saw how much peace he was finding, and how much self-discovery he was enjoying. He even seemed more 'in tune' with the Universe in general and instead of just talking about it, I saw some real changes taking place in his life and his attitude. He didn't seem to harbor any ill will toward his past and he looked forward to his future, despite some of the difficulties he was still facing. I wanted that for myself. I'd always been religious in the sense that I believed in God but I'd never been very spiritual, and I've since learned the two are very different. That was something I had to find a way to understand. At first it didn't make any sense to me, but I was desperately seeking a way to come to terms with everything I'd been through and where I needed to go from that point – and why. Now it was really up to me. I could step up and take responsibility and keep moving forward, or I could let myself fall back into the old habits that had gotten me nowhere. I didn't want to do that. I knew on some level I'd broken the pattern I'd been following for so long, but whether it would stay broken or find a way to repair itself, and what it really meant overall for the course of my future and an understanding of my past, was still a mystery to me.

At that point I'd still not heard the terms 'relationship addict,' or 'love addict,' or anything along those lines. I knew about stalkers and things like that – people who were obsessed with a particular movie star – but that was as far as I'd gone with thinking about that kind of issue. It just didn't seem like it had any relevance to me. I saw myself as a person with depression and anxiety who'd been through an incredible run of bad luck where men were concerned. I didn't see myself as 'addicted,' and I didn't see the problems I was having with other relationships, like the relationship with my daughter or my parents, or even the few friends I had. It seemed normal to me, because I didn't know any better. I wasn't aware of any other way to be. I did feel like I had to make a few changes, because I wasn't where I wanted to be in my personal life or my career or my finances, and as my depression started to lift I started to become more aware of that. It was a struggle to see the problems I was really facing and to realize I had created most of them, and it wasn't something that happened in a day. It would have happened faster but I fought it because I didn't know what else to do. I wanted the change, but only if *I* didn't have to change to get it.

I'm not sure if that makes sense anywhere but in my own head, but I'll try to explain it. I wanted things to be different because I didn't like the way they'd been going over the last thirty years of my life or so, ever since I was a kid. On the other hand, I knew what this life was like. It might not have been great, but there was a pattern and a method to it, and it had a certain comfort level I'd come to expect. Changing would mean stepping out of that comfort level – likely for good – and doing things differently. It was both exciting and scary, and I couldn't decide which of those two emotions would win the day. Ultimately I wanted to just keep doing things the way I'd been doing them all along and have everything else around me change to provide more benefit to my life. It wasn't going to happen. Of course it wasn't. And I think I knew that deep down inside, but I wasn't willing to admit it yet. I still hoped some miracle would come along and change things. But what I was slowly coming to realize was that miracle had already come along in the form of Klaus and his German music, and now I had to learn to be my own miracle for the future.

Unlike an alcoholic who makes a choice to remain sober and takes all the alcohol out of the house to help with that commitment, there was only so much I could do with my relationships. I couldn't become a hermit, because I had responsibilities to others. In addition, I would never learn anything valuable by continuing to run away from my problems. It was good I had no husband or boyfriend. That was a start toward a different kind of life. I had a daughter, though, and friends and parents who I couldn't just simply ignore. Because of that, recovery was something I had to find my way with, based on trial and error. I turned to spirituality mostly because of Klaus, but also because I had a yearning to do more and have more and *be* more than I was. I was happier than I'd been in a long time, but I still wasn't what I would consider 'at peace' or 'content' with myself and my life. I wanted that peace. It was a strong desire of mine to feel I was content. The only times I truly had that feeling was when I was listening to music. That was a wonderful respite from the way I felt during most other times, especially when I felt anxious or panicky or down and depressed, but I wanted to take that peace and contentment with me when I turned off the CD player or the iPod. I'd forgotten what it was like to feel that way in my day to day life, but I knew I couldn't wait any longer for the memory to come back to me. I had to go out and get it myself. And so I did.

I started on my journey in what I consider to be a most unusual way. I mean…German hip-hop music? Really? When I tell my story to people they look at me like I've just told them something crazy. They either think it's the stupidest thing they've ever heard or the coolest thing they've ever heard – there doesn't seem to be much middle ground. I don't blame them. If it hadn't actually happened to me I'm not sure how I'd feel about it either. Everyone has something that works for them, even if they haven't yet located it. It's one of those things most people have to look for – I was fortunate that it fell into my lap, and looking for it wasn't necessary, but it sure did take me a long time to get there! If I'd gone looking I might have found it much more rapidly, but every time I started to make a change or venture out of the pattern of life I'd created I'd get scared – or my parents would balk at the idea – so I'd just retreat back into my shell and stop mentioning it, secretly dying a little bit inside each time. At night I'd dream of being somewhere else, some*one* else, with a totally different life. What would that be like? I really wanted to know, yet I was afraid to take the steps to find out.

When I finally decided change wasn't going to come to me and I had to do something different for myself and for Karyn, I spent a lot of time in introspection. I don't even know why I did it that way. It just seemed like the right thing to do – be quiet and still and wait for that little voice inside to offer some direction. Now that I didn't have a man in my life I had more time to myself, and I used some of that time to try to figure out what had been going on that had caused so much trouble. As I started to explore my own psyche more fully, I began realizing the pattern I'd been in for so long: one relationship after another, and no real love. I got married for the sake of getting married. I needed to feel like I belonged to someone. I never married for love. Never. Not true and lasting love, anyway. I married for the idea of being in love, hoping that it would work out this time. I wanted to show my parents I was a real person with a real life, worthy of their respect. I wanted them to love me, and even though they insisted they did I still had a hard time acknowledging that. I've only recently come to a real understanding that I've had their love and respect all my life, regardless of what I've done right or wrong in their eyes.

The love and respect I really needed *was my own*, and that was something no one else could give me. I had to give it to myself, which was much easier said than done. I wasn't sure where I should even start. It wasn't as simple as just thinking good thoughts – I had to find a justification for everything that had taken place so I could begin to move past it. It was the way I handled everything in my life – justifying it logically so it made sense to me. While playing around on the computer late one night and not really thinking about much, I decided to do some research for a friend who was struggling with some compulsions. He was trying to help himself but he needed to do more – go to meetings, maybe seek some therapy – to get better. I was worried about him, and wanted to see him get better. I started searching for sites regarding 'sex addiction' and that pulled up sites on other types of related addictions – like love and relationship addiction.

As soon as I saw the words on the screen I felt an instant and intense interest in them. Something just clicked. I tried to ignore it, because it would imply that the problem had been – and still was – mine, not anyone else's. I finished the research for my friend and went on to do some other things, but my mind kept coming back to the 'relationship addiction' term. I felt it was important to me, but I was still in so much denial. I was pretty happy, at least on the surface, for the first time in a long time, and the last thing I wanted was to sabotage that feeling by delving into areas that might change my views on things or my understanding of them. The denial was safe and secure.

A few sleepless hours later I found myself in front of the computer again, typing 'relationship addiction' into the search engine and taking a deep breath. When I hit the search button I knew what I was doing was going to affect me, and there would be no going back. It was a deliberate action as the result of a gut feeling, and I'd come to trust in those a little more. I was still a skeptic, but I was moving toward a less pessimistic outlook on the strangeness that was starting to happen all around me with increasing frequency. I'd been having these little 'revelation experiences,' what Klaus had dubbed 'a-ha moments,' ever since I started on my own spiritual journey – or maybe I'd been having them all along and was only now beginning to understand what they meant. Since I was trying to find something that would help me understand my life and why it had gone the way it had, I was forcing myself to be more open to those little moments and gut feelings – trying them out and seeing where they led.

The one that kept leading me toward change had led me to research relationship addiction, and research it I did. When I really commit to something, truly and deeply, I don't do things half-assed. I *studied*. It wasn't good enough for me to just know *what*. I had to know *how, why,* and all the other issues that surrounded the main question. Of course, I didn't understand everything right away. There was no 'Eureka!' moment of perfect clarity as I read about the problem and its symptoms. It was more like slowly coming around to an acceptance of something you really didn't want to face in the first place. No one wants to admit there's something wrong with them, and I was no exception. I didn't want to say I was an addict – of any kind. It seemed weak. Until the moment some days later when I finally truly accepted that I was a relationship addict, I don't think I ever really *understood* that addiction was *real*. There's a definite difference between *knowing* something and *understanding* something. At that time, I still saw drug and alcohol addicts as weak-minded, and food addicts as weaker still. Why didn't they just *stop?* But if I could be addicted to *relationships*...to *people*...well, I had no room at all to judge others, now did I?

My acceptance that I was, and am, a relationship addict changed my perspective on life. I didn't look at things the same way after that. Just as music changed my outlook on life to a more positive one, my acceptance of who and what I was changed my perspective to a more understanding and introspective one. I guess you could say I went from being depressed and shallow to being happy and deep, but that's about the most simplistic way it could ever be stated. It was a lot more significant than that, and it took a while. Even once understanding dawns, change is not always automatic. People have to *want* to change – and I did – but they have to also understand *how* to change, or be willing to learn how, and that was something I hadn't found myself to be capable of just yet. Still, just being able to say I was a relationship addict – even if it was only out loud to myself when no one else was around – was a tremendous step in the right direction. Once I was able to do that, I was able to go deeper into my own personal analysis of my life, and I started to see the relationship patterns I had succumbed to more clearly than I ever had before. When you're no longer trying to hide from yourself it's amazing how clearly you begin to see things.

When I married for the first time, I did it because I wanted to fit in and get a head start on a 'real' life. I didn't see I was doing something that was designed to fail. I didn't see I wasn't in love, or that the volatility of the relationship I'd had with Daniel wasn't a good precursor to a marriage. Actually, I *did* see it, deep down, but I ignored it and I rationalized it away. I was so desperate to get married because I thought I'd be accepted by society that way. I shouldn't have done it, or at the least I should have waited longer. I could have made sure he was the right person instead of just telling myself he was. I could have taken the time to determine what I actually wanted from life and from a relationship. I could have given us both some time to grow up. Who really knows what they want at seventeen anyway? But I knew I wanted the attention...and I'm not even sure why. It's not like my parents ignored me – they basically lavished attention on me, to the point of it being too much sometimes. You'd have thought I would've wanted *less* attention, not more. I think some of the problems I faced in school and how I never really fit in with anyone had a lot to do with why I wanted to get married so young.

Not only did I feel like I would 'fit in' with the married lifestyle, but I felt like I'd be more respected, and respect was something I'd never gotten from my peers. Even being smart didn't get me respected by others in my age group, because none of them really cared much about that. Friends, and later boys and cars, were what mattered to them. Being smart just got me labeled 'book worm' and 'teacher's pet' and all kinds of far nastier names. I wanted everyone to see me as a real person with a real life. I thought getting married would do that, because it would make me an adult, and adults don't treat each other that way, right? Right. Sure. Adults can be just as mean, they just find other ways to do it. Snide comments about various things. Snickers behind your back. Being overlooked for promotions or shut out of the after work get-togethers on Friday nights. Marrying young didn't get me any respect. A few younger people thought it was cool, but for the most part people just thought I was stupid. The comment I got most often was 'Are you pregnant?' No, I wasn't, but I couldn't seem to make people understand that. When I got married it was with the idea I would then be treated as an adult, but adults only thought I was a dumb teenager who didn't know what I was doing.

When I married for the second time, I thought Tyler was so different from Daniel! He seemed so sweet and kind and good natured – and he was easy to control. He did what I told him to do, almost always without question. I was a little bit older when I entered into that marriage, and I thought because of that I was a lot wiser. I figured I could do a better job and make a better choice this time. I still thought I would be seen as an adult and taken more seriously. Since it didn't happen the first time I don't know why I thought it would happen the second time, but I loved being able to say 'my fiancé,' or 'my husband.' I felt so grown up, and it identified me as a person who was allegedly loved by others. I mattered to someone. Someone thought I was good enough to *marry*…and it was great when strangers would admire my ring or ask when I was getting married or how long I'd been married. It put me in the limelight again and gave me that attention I felt I deserved. It was an act. A desperate attempt to live a 'normal' life so others would see how good I was at it. Except I wasn't good at it. I could fake it for a while, and then I was bored and restless and making trouble in my marriage and moving on.

I saw that looming pattern on some level when Tyler and I split up. I'd planned that divorce for a while before it took place. I remember stroking Karyn's tiny head and wispy hair when she was just a baby and telling her pretty soon it would be just her and me…and soon it was, because I made it so. I effectively found a way to justify everything I was doing and make a mountain out of a molehill for anything Tyler did. In my own little world, I could do no wrong. That was an act, too. I *knew* I wasn't doing things right, but I was so far in denial it wasn't even funny by the time Tyler and I divorced. And then I turned around and did it three more times! Even a child could've seen there was a pattern to my problems. I got married because I was lonely and bored and wanted some drama and excitement in my life, and then when I decided it wasn't fun anymore I got divorced. Unfortunately, I didn't learn my lesson from that for some reason – maybe I was just too stubborn – so I continued to follow that pattern, telling myself it was the person I married, not the marriage itself, that was the problem.

Ridiculous, I know, but that's what addiction is all about. You *don't* see what you're doing, and how you're hurting yourself and others. You're desperate to get your 'fix,' and my fix was marriage – or more specifically the time between finding a new man and turning that encounter into a wedding. The actual married life I could've mostly done without. I'm a friendly person, but I'm not a *social* person. I love to visit and be around people for a little while, but then I want them to leave so I can have my own space and be left alone. Married life of course doesn't give you that unless your spouse travels almost all the time. I knew this before I got married, each and every time, but I thought it would be different that time. The one thing I simply cannot do is explain to you why I thought that. Part of it had to do with the person I married – if I just get the right one I won't mind him being around all the time. The truth of the matter was I would've minded no matter who it was. It could've been the 'perfect' person for me, and I still would've found a reason to mess things up. I would've sabotaged the marriage, where I might not have sabotaged the relationship if we'd not married – but I couldn't understand the concept of not marrying. It made no sense to me.

It was one of those concepts that you hear, but you don't understand. I have the same problem with things like Algebra. I see the equation and you can explain to me how to do it, but I'm not good at doing it myself. It doesn't make any sense to me, and it doesn't seem to matter how it's presented. It's like there's a block in my brain that prevents me from 'getting' that concept. The same was true of the idea of dating someone indefinitely. Concept block. A lot of men don't want to just date forever. They're either looking for a one-nighter or other casual fling, or they're looking to marry and settle down and have children – but I'm sure not all men are like that. There are certainly some out there who'd be happy with a long-term girlfriend.

After my second marriage ended I insisted that kind of relationship was what I was looking for and I never wanted to get married again, and yet I turned around and got married thrice more anyway. I didn't seem to be able to reconcile what I *said* with what I *did.* I wish I could say 'I did this because…' and give a real, valid, understandable reason, but I can't do that. Any of you who have addiction issues or know someone who does will understand my inability to give what would be considered a 'real' reason. You don't really know why you do things, sometimes. If you could break your addiction you probably would, but you don't know how. Or you might not want to break your addiction because you're used to it – you feel safe; it's routine. Sometimes you either don't know you have an addiction problem or don't think your problem is serious enough to warrant doing anything about it. You may feel confused and conflicted, and not understand why all these kinds of things are happening to you. You may not *want* to understand why these things are happening to you, because that would mean admitting you have a problem – something wrong with *you,* not the people around you. It's frightening.

I was scared. No, actually I was terrified. I didn't know what acceptance and change was ultimately going to do to me and how it might re-shape my life. I didn't like the unknown and I wanted and needed to be in control, always. Of course that's actually impossible, but when I was in such denial about my addiction I was also in denial about my ability to control my own destiny – I still believed it was me, not God, who was handling everything that was going on in my life. I didn't have a lot of use for God during the time period between the end of my last marriage and the discovery of the truth about my relationship patterns and my addiction – mostly because I didn't think He was doing enough to rectify my situation. I was spoiled and I wanted everything handed to me, instead of having to work for it. I felt everyone *owed* me, including God. I still feel a little uncomfortable admitting that but God knows what's in my heart, so He's already aware of it. It's no shock to Him. Essentially, I was still playing the victim, and this was true in my relationships with my family members and friends as well as my past husbands and boyfriends.

No matter what was going on in my life, I found some reason to have some drama. Either something was going terribly right or something was going extremely wrong. I didn't like the middle ground because I wasn't getting attention, either in the form of sympathy or praise. It didn't matter to me which one I was getting, as long as it was one or the other. As I got older, and kept making the same choices over and over again, the sympathy I got from my family and friends started to wane. People were getting tired of my antics, I'm sure, and since none of them knew about relationship addiction, it wasn't like they could stage some kind of intervention and get me some help. I don't know if it would've done any good even if they had tried that. Until I was willing to truly and completely admit I was the one causing this, nothing anyone else could've said or done would've changed the way I was living my life.

Once I accepted the truth of my addiction, I began to work on my understanding of it, and that became a spiritual issue. I'm not so sure I even meant for it to end up that way. My parents weren't spiritual people – at least not outwardly where I could see it and be shaped by it growing up – and Klaus was the only spiritual friend I really had. Max developed a much more spiritual outlook later on, but his choices about belief were quite a bit different from mine, so they didn't really help me. The more I looked at my life, the more I realized that Klaus' idea of spirituality was quite a bit different from mine, too. I couldn't really get any help from him, either. I had to develop my own concept of it, which was made more difficult by the fact that I lacked direction when it came to that issue. I didn't know *how* to be spiritual, or whether one thing worked better than another. I was raised to think things through, and I couldn't do that with this, because thinking and planning wasn't what spirituality was about. It was a personal, individual thing that's different for everyone. I would have to find my own way.

Since I was raised a conservative Christian, I had some real issues with 'being spiritual' in the first place, and I had to work through them before I could do anything else. Not only did I not know how to do it, but I was also uncertain about whether it was blasphemous. If I thought positive thoughts and admired nature and meditated, would that be like praying? Or would it be like worshipping false idols? I wasn't sure, and I was conflicted about what to do next. But I also knew I needed to find a different way to look at the world consistently so I could keep my depression and anxiety at bay and make sure the relationship pattern I had finally gotten away from stayed broken. I couldn't listen to music every waking minute so I sought other – legal and moral – ways to get that same feeling of peace and contentment; that feeling that absolutely everything was right with the world. I went back to praying, but I didn't say the same rote words I had learned. Instead, I actually *prayed.* I said what I wanted to say, asked for what I felt I needed, said 'thank you' for the things I was really thankful for. I just *talked* to God, like you'd talk to a friend you trusted. I suppose it was unorthodox and it felt really strange at first, but it started to make me feel better, and that was something that praying hadn't been able to do for me in a very long time.

I was feeling closer to God, but I wasn't feeling closer to myself...and my gut was telling me that was one of the most important issues I had to work on. I had to learn to love and care about and respect myself. What happened wasn't my fault, just like it's not the alcoholic's fault he or she used to drink. Addiction is a sickness...a disease; it's a problem with brain chemistry and how a person's life has been shaped. It's not done to deliberately inflict pain on oneself or others, but too many people who are recovering addicts of any kind are awash in a sea of shame and misery and guilt. They feel like everything that's gone poorly in the lives of anyone they've ever been around was somehow their fault. I know I felt that way, too. Getting over the guilt was something I knew wouldn't come easily to me. I had guilt about my childhood, about the way I treated my grandmother in her battle with Alzheimer's, about my marriages, and about the way I interacted with my friends and family, even as an adult. How was I just supposed to let all that go? Who would I be if I wasn't the innocent victim or the guilty party? If I didn't deserve sympathy or if I wasn't the martyr? Who would I be if I was just *me*?

With the asking of those kinds of questions I began to realize why I wasn't getting anywhere with prayer or with my spiritual journey or with the rest of my life – I didn't know who I was. I'd always been someone's child and/or someone's wife. I identified myself by who I was in relation to the people around me, not by who I really was on the inside, as a person apart from others. I didn't feel like I had ever, really, just 'been me.' Who was I, truly, deep down on the inside? If you stripped away all the pain and the anxiety and the depression and the addiction and the other problems I faced throughout my life, what was left? What did *that person* want? Who was she, and what could she become? There was still time.

For a while, I went through a stage of serious guilt. I wanted to find just about every person I'd ever met and apologize to them, even if I couldn't remember wronging them. I realized what an impossible task this would be, so I did what I could. Some people might think that was silly, and that's fine too. I'd always been taught what goes around comes around, but I never paid much attention to that statement. Now I thought I might give it a try. Mostly, I just wanted to see if it was true. Would my life really improve if I started living it differently?

With as many little 'a-ha moments' as I'd started to have I don't know why I was surprised by the way things happened, but things *did* start to improve. For every nice thing I did, it seemed like I got something back. It might have been something small, or it might have been something bigger, but it was always something. If I gave money to a homeless person I'd get an email from a potential client wanting some work done, always adding up to considerably more than the amount I gave. If I was kind to someone in the grocery store I might find some loose change, or someone would do something nice for me I wasn't expecting. Soon I was looking for nice things to do for others...and it wasn't even greed – it was honest curiosity about what would happen next. If I did X, would I get Y...or would I get Z? I just didn't know, and it was almost like a game to me. I began to share my observations with my daughter and with Klaus, and then later with my mother when I realized she was interested in it as well. My father found some of the anecdotes amusing and strange, but I'm not sure he *believed* in them the way the rest of us did. It was exciting, and I began to see some strange and wonderful things taking place in both my life and my attitude.

My daughter had come a long way, too. I enrolled her in a private Christian school and she excelled, flying through her studies and making high grades. It was seriously impressive, and she was so happy she didn't have to go to public school and be harassed ever again. It further helped her outlook on life and stopped her from being so cynical about human beings overall. It didn't turn her into a giggling, bouncy person, but she'd never been that way. She was – and still is – quiet and serious, much like me. I didn't want or need her to be someone else. I just wanted her to be happy and content and at peace, and she was working toward finding those things. I was trying to help her along with helping myself, but something that works for one person doesn't always work for another person. I could give her suggestions and offer advice, but her own spiritual journey was something she would have to ultimately go through alone. It's one of those things no one can do for you. You have to wander around in the dark, trying to find your way, until you come out into the light on the other side – much like the way many people go through their entire lives. I was one of those wandering, blundering people not so very long ago.

The kinds of things that helped me break my relationship pattern and started me on a path toward a lot more joy and happiness and peace might not be your cup of tea. They might not do anything for you. It's fine if they don't – but *something* will. Even if you aren't sure what to do next, there *is* something out there that will resonate with your soul. When you find it, it'll just click, and you'll *know* it's the right thing. Don't question that knowing. I could have done much more to help myself earlier in my life had I simply *listened* to myself – to that gut feeling, that internal voice we all have – instead of listening to everyone else and trying to please them. I don't mean to say you shouldn't ever do something to please another person or you should be completely focused on pleasing only yourself. But being unhappy with yourself doesn't help you to help others. If you're happy with yourself, you'll be a lot more interested in doing things for other people. But those things will be on your terms, and they won't make you feel bad or guilty by compromising what you ultimately feel is the right path for your life.

People who struggle with relationship addiction often fall into their relationship patterns very early on in their lives. Much of what they learn in childhood shapes what it is they see as important in later life, and their addiction distorts those views. In other words, a mentally healthy person with no addiction or behavioral health issues wouldn't have the same type of understanding of his or her life and the way it works as someone struggling with relationship addiction or anxiety or both. There are definite differences as to how all people see the world, of course, but there are even stronger differences between people with addiction problems and those who do not deal with these kinds of issues. Because so many things shape a person's life a relationship addict – or any other type of addict – can't usually pinpoint just one specific issue as a trigger point for his or her problems. For example, my own relationship pattern came from several things:

- Wanting to be accepted by my parents and not feeling like anything I did for them was good enough to keep them happy. No matter how much love they gave me I always felt like I never deserved it. I kept waiting to see when they were going to change their minds or get tired of me and every year that went past made me more nervous about when that change was coming, instead of more sure it would not.
- Wanting to be accepted by society but continually being teased and harassed by other children at school. I didn't fit in. I was too smart and too adult, and

because of that people in my own age group thought I was a freak, or thought I was stupid. The kinds of games and activities I liked weren't 'normal' for my age, but there were no outside-the-family adults to interact with, so I was stuck.

- Wanting to feel like and be treated like an adult but not understanding that marriage was not the way to obtain that. It could've been done through other measures, or it could've been avoided until I simply 'grew into it,' but I didn't see any of that. I only saw marriage as a way for people to see me as a grown-up human being.

- Wanting the long-term love my parents had with each other but not waiting to be sure the person I 'loved' was actually the right person for me. I never really thought about the 'right' person – I just needed a person. I would take him and turn him into what it was I needed, rather than waste any time hunting for someone who already had the right qualities. That seemed like too much work and too much effort, not to mention the fact that it might take a while.

If I had gone about solving my concerns correctly, my life would've been drastically different, but the addiction problems got in the way. A person with my basic childhood experiences but no addiction or anxiety problems would've been much more likely to already feel accepted by his or her parents, and would've been unconcerned as to whether society accepted him or her or not. He or she would also probably have been more well-adjusted and therefore more accepted overall. In addition, that person would've likely had more patience with the speed and course of life and not been in such a hurry for adulthood through a relationship, knowing being treated like an adult would come with time and would be better served with things like education and work experience. Finding that long-term love would only come from waiting for the *right* person, not just *any* person, which would be something our fictional individual would be willing to do.

Naturally, everyone makes mistakes. If I'd gotten married the first time, gotten divorced, and not remarried...or not remarried until some years later and then stayed married that second time, I'd count that first marriage as a mistake. When you've done something five times in a row, though, it's hard to just say 'oops!' and shrug it off. It wears on you, and it wears on the people around you. After a while everyone starts rolling their eyes every time you mention a name that sounds like it might belong to someone of the opposite sex, and it makes you feel bad and conflicted. I went through periods of 'I'm so stupid!' and periods of 'I'll show *them*!' Most of the time I was somewhere in the middle, or trying to be in both places at once, until I felt like I might just break apart. The fact that I kept doing the same things over and over but never saw a pattern despite my intelligence level is good proof of the insidiousness of addiction and how it can steal your life away while you're not paying attention. You don't even realize it's taking place until you come out of it, and some people never make it that far. This is especially true with drug and alcohol addiction, both of which have a nasty habit of killing people, but people can get 'stuck' in relationship addiction, too, and there's no guarantee they won't die from it.

People can get deadly diseases from compulsions and addictions regarding promiscuity, or they can be killed at the hands of a jealous and violent spouse they stay with out of fear or the belief they aren't good enough to deserve someone better. They could even die from the hygiene problems of someone – like my last husband and his lack of cleanliness making me so sick all the time. There are thousands of ways to die, and someone with anxiety like me doesn't really like to be reminded of that, but it's important. People don't think about how *dangerous* relationship addiction might actually be, especially in the long term. They don't take it seriously, even though they should. Raising awareness is important so people can realize what's going on, why they might be doing what they're doing, or how to help someone they love and care about.

People in the middle of their problems rarely see those problems. They only see what they want to see – it's like they've got blinders on. It's amazing how much a human being can ignore, or how many things they can rationalize away when they don't want to take responsibility for what they're doing or admit that they might have a problem. I did it for so long, and I'm sure a lot of other people with all different kinds of addictions do the same thing. I know I'm not alone in this one. They think, like I did, that whatever they're doing has to be right because they're the ones doing it. It's their life story, they're the one starring in it, and so it has to be everyone else who's messing things up. The blame game was a big deal with me until I accepted my addiction and what I was doing to myself and others – but when you stop blaming others it's very important you don't start blaming yourself. There's a difference between doing something deliberately and doing something because you're wrestling with an addiction.

The hardest thing for me to comprehend when I stopped blaming other people was that it wasn't my fault, either. There is no 'at fault' where addiction is concerned. Things simply are what they are. The most important thing is realizing the problem and taking steps to keep it at bay in the future, not trying to determine what you should feel guilty about from the past. If you think back through your life and make peace with the choices you made because you understand your addiction now, and then you move on, that's totally different from torturing yourself by constantly reminding yourself of the things you chose that were 'wrong.' Sometimes, you start out to do one thing and you end up doing something else. I've tried to look back on my life and make peace with it several times, and I've gotten a lot better at it, but there are still things I feel guilty about, or things I wish I'd done differently. I still sometimes feel like I've wasted a lot of time, even though I know no time is really 'wasted.' There's a purpose in everything we do, even when we're doing nothing at all, but it's hard to accept that sometimes.

Feeling guilty won't change anything, because I can't undo what's been done. Even if I'd had a marriage or two annulled instead of getting divorced, the marriage would've still existed. Just because the court would've wiped the slate clean doesn't mean the time I spent with that person would've ceased to exist. It also doesn't mean God would've forgotten I made a promise and then broke it. That was a big worry for me. I know the Bible says some things about divorce, and they aren't comments in favor of the activity. I also know Jesus forgave a woman who said she'd been married five times. The issue of forgiveness and whether I had it or not was a big one for me for a long time. It was another one of those things I had to learn to let go of. If God wasn't willing to forgive me even though I'd asked Him to, there wasn't anything I could do about that. It all goes back to not being able to take back what I've already done, and I worked at moving past the past, because finding out what was wrong with me and then living the rest of my life feeling guilty about it wasn't what I wanted to do. I wanted to *live*, not just exist, and once I saw some of the things I tried actually making a difference I was determined to continue them and add more to the mix – anything to feel totally and completely human.

I moved deeper into the spiritual aspect of my life and just slowly felt my way along, using what worked for me and discarding the rest. I didn't have a choice if I wanted to recover – I had to help myself. I'd been given the tools I needed to use but it was up to me to get those tools out on a regular basis and continue to work with them. Tools that don't get used get rusty and don't do anybody any good. Even if I had gone to a traditional therapist and paid a lot of money to be told what was wrong with me, he or she still wouldn't have been able to change me or my behavior. I had to do that myself. It wasn't easy. I'm not going to lie and say it was, or gloss it over and say you can 'fix' your addiction problem in a couple of days – all you need is some foreign music, some prayer, and a little willpower. I wish it was that easy for everyone. I wish it'd been that easy for me. Fortunately, it's possible to recover, it's possible to forgive yourself and others, and it's possible to live a full and complete life again, no matter what you've been through in the past.

Even if you don't believe that right now, or even if you don't believe in yourself any more, you can still get through this, just like I did. At my lowest point I really did want to die, but yet I was so terrified of it, as well. I was stuck, and one of my favorite authors, Robert Fulghum, once made a comment about someone like that in one of his tales. He said the man he was talking about was stuck, and he thought that 'getting unstuck' and 'coming unglued' were the same thing. I had the same problem. I could identify with that statement. Strongly. I had to change but I didn't know what change would bring, and I didn't know what to do next. My changes came mostly out of anger and desperation – out of simply being tired of existing the way I was. It would've been nice if I could've 'learned my lesson' a lot faster, but some people never learn it at all. I was actually quite fortunate to have a chance to change my ways and my behavior; to recognize my addiction for what it was before it became any more destructive to my life or to the lives of other people around me.

Through patience and perseverance, and through sheer force of will, I kept working on it. I thought positive things. I meditated. I said affirmations out loud each morning. I prayed fervently. I practiced breathing. I started taking walks again, and when I did I looked around – I mean really *looked* at what was around me. I'd been so busy feeling bad I hadn't really seen all the beauty in my life and in my local area. I was five minutes from the beach. Everything around me was green and alive. There were neighbors to wave at. I hadn't even really noticed. The joy and beauty of life was going on all around me. I feel bad that I missed so much of it, but I feel blessed there is still so much of it for me to see. I know it's there now, and I won't overlook it again. I can't allow myself to slip back into the old relationship and anxiety and depression patterns I used to take comfort in even while I was miserable. I owe it to myself and my family and friends, and to the people I will meet and know in the future, to remind myself each day of who I am and what I'm worth – both to God and to myself. You owe it to yourself to do that, as well.

What I Did **Right**
- Was willing to let myself change even though I knew it wouldn't be easy.
- Gained enough bravery to go out and find my happiness on my own.
- Really thought about what I needed to do to improve my life and keep it moving forward.

- Discovered I wouldn't feel like I had the respect and love of other people until I had respect and love for myself.
- Became willing to do the work to find out the root of my problem.
- Stopped judging others as I came to understand that other addicts were not weak.
- Really analyzed why I did what I did, so I could come to an understanding of it and get some closure on my past.
- Learned to let go of the guilt and the shame.
- Started treating myself and others the way I should have been – with kindness and respect.
- Let myself become open to new ideas and new experiences, even if they're a little scary sometimes.

What To Look For
- Understanding you need to change even if it's difficult.
- Discovering that you're willing to work on your difficulties and find the root of them.
- A desire to finally let go of the shame and guilt you're carrying.
- Opening yourself up to new ideas, even if there's some fear mixed in with them.
- Wanting to treat people better, and understanding why it's important.
- Wanting to treat *yourself* better because you see that you have worth.
- A willingness to analyze your past so you can have peace in the present and get ready for the future.

What The Therapist Says

This chapter reaches a point in the recovery process that is often highly uncomfortable for a codependent relationship addict. I had mentioned before how difficult it is for the addict to face those behavioral patterns which constitute the addiction. But beyond recognition lie two more steps, steps that are often even harder to get through. The first is acknowledgment: the admission of the sufferer not just of the presence of the addiction pattern but of the fact that he or she *is* a relationship addict. On the surface there may be little distinction between admitting to addictive behavior and actually being an addict, yet in terms of our subconscious these two concepts differ greatly. By admitting that we not only engage in certain behaviors but that we are definitely addicted to them we acknowledge not only the problem, we also admit to our helplessness in the light of it.

Following this milestone is another, even more arduous step. After acknowledging the problem, then admitting to our helplessness, we now have to reach a level of acceptance of the situation. Since most codependency sufferers are already burdened with a low level of self-acceptance it is easy to comprehend how difficult this step is to them. Yet one must not confuse the concepts of "accepting" with "being happy with." We can admit and accept that a certain situation exists, even though we most definitely dislike that same situation. Acceptance is simply the removal of any last bits of self-denial or rationalization. Once the relationship addict has reached this level, the door is now open for the active recovery process to begin.

I have already mentioned affirmations, creative expression, and support groups as good starting points in beginning to fill the internal void created by the addict's low sense of self-worth. This chapter touches on another recovery aspect, which has been shown to be of extreme help not only in codependence and relationship addiction, but in most addictive conditions or disorders linked to deficiencies in self-esteem. This aspect deals with spirituality. In the context used here spirituality should not be confused with religious practice. The former is meant to express a deeply felt personal connection with, for lack of a better word, a "Higher Power," while the later defines the practicing of a certain religious denomination or creed. Through this distinction one can discern that the two concepts do not necessarily depend on each other. One can feel a deep, personal connection to one's Higher Power without following particular religious rites just as one can engage in a number of religious practices without ever having felt that personal connection.

This differentiation often distresses certain individuals, as the most common context in which we are told we can achieve the spiritual connection is religious practice. And it is true that many people do achieve their spirituality by following a specific religion. Historically speaking, the most common path used to achieve spiritual experiences has probably been through religious practice. Just as these two concepts are not identical they are also not mutually exclusive. But it is important to understand that one does not guarantee the presence of the other.

So what is spirituality? The opinions as to what constitutes spirituality, both personal and professional, are vast and varied. A good way to understanding the concept is to determine what benefits people have described from it. Most individuals who consider themselves to be spiritual state that they believe and trust in "something greater" than themselves. This belief, in turn, supplies them not only with an unconditional trust, but also reduces their subconscious need to exert perfect control over their lives for fear of impending disaster. Another important aspect common to the idea of a "Higher Power" is that it represents a source of unconditional love and acceptance. To the spiritual person, his "Higher Power" will see him as worthy and lovable even when he has made a mistake. As such, the "Higher Power" becomes the external source for validation a codependent can always count on, a source that is not only unconditional but potentially infinite in capacity.

When viewed rationally this would make spiritual contact the perfect remedy for any addiction based on codependence and low self-worth. If the "Higher Power" represents an unlimited supply of validation, no matter how one behaves, than it would, speaking hypothetically, serve as the only viable source to fill that equally unlimited internal void that the lack of self-esteem creates.

The next obvious question would be how one can obtain this "perfect fit;" this spiritual experience that can serve as the solution to the subconscious ego-deficiencies obvious in codependent relationship addiction. The answer to that is sadly a bit more complex than just taking a pill or making the decision to "become spiritual." Just as relationship addiction and codependence are learned behaviors and attitudes, so a spiritual attitude has to be practiced and trained in order to become effective. Again, many people become confused at this point as to how one practices spirituality in order to become "good" at it. There are a number of different strategies one can employ, including engaging in religious activities. Yet all of these will probably share a few common denominators.

One common aspect of spiritual practices, and I do mean "practice" as in "having to practice," has to do with the believer trying to give over his or her worries, fears, even hopes and desires to his or her Higher Power with the intent of removing any related anxieties or disappointments from the mind. The practices as to how this letting go process is achieved are varied and numerous. They can range from simple prayer – asking the Higher Power to remove all the worries from one's life – to meditative visualization where the practitioner visually imagines handing over all the things that bother him/her to whatever form the Higher Power takes. Some individuals pick up sticks and stones and then imagine putting their fears and desires into them before throwing them away, thereby symbolically throwing away all those needs the subconscious does not want to let go of.

Another component related to this has to do with trying to quiet one's own mind, especially in regard to obsessive thoughts and worries. Again, prayers and mantras that focus the practitioner's mind away from internal thoughts and toward the prayer can be used for that. Deep meditation or breathing exercises that carry a person's attention away from worries and concerns are also useful and can be learned independently through books and audio materials as well as through teachers. Other techniques involve focusing on the "here and now" rather than worrying about the future or regretting the past. Such "here and now" exercises often try to channel a person's attention to things he or she can physically sense, things that can be positively appreciated.

Appreciation and positive focus are other concepts often utilized in spiritual pursuits as well as unrelated recovery practices. They aim at getting a person to immediately focus his attention on something positive, as soon as the mind begins to belabor sad, negative, and self-defeating thoughts. These positive things can be positive aspects of our own selves we can remind ourselves of whenever we engage in self-deprecation. Especially when we feel we have done something very poorly, we can practice self-talk that acknowledges both our mistake as well as the fact that doing something poorly or badly does not make us "bad." An example of this would be saying, "My boss said I never do any good work, *nevertheless*, I am still a lovable and worthwhile person." In this example the word "nevertheless" is the one that allows our subconscious to separate the negative external feedback from our sense of self-worth. Again, these thought exercises have to be practiced whenever we become aware of our negative self-talk in order to affect long-term change in our attitudes.

But refocusing on something positive whenever a situation causes us to feel poorly about ourselves can also be done using our external senses. When having a bad day, filled with ideas of low self-esteem, external factors that would normally make us happier, like a sunny day or listening to a nice piece of music, can be used to lift our emotional response. The only thing required is an effort to focus on the appreciation of the external sensory stimulus. This can be accomplished by telling ourselves, either in our minds or even verbally, how much we enjoy whatever external thing we use as the center of our appreciation. Since the subconscious listens to experience, and both the external focus of appreciation and the self-talk are experiential, it will be more likely to internalize these positives than if we simply tried to rationalize our negative thoughts away. Experience and practice are the keys.

Chapter 11: The Journey Continues

So, who am I now? I'm – finally – just me. Michielle DJ Beck. My friends call me Michi...and I'm a recovering relationship addict. Am I still sometimes ashamed of my past? Sure. Do I still sometimes feel guilty? Yes, of course I do. I think those are normal human reactions to the kinds of past experiences I've had. I worry about what I've put people through and what I've put myself through. I get nervous about all the strained relationships and I feel like I should apologize again, even though I've been told it's OK numerous times by family and friends. Still, though, I'm glad to feel some emotions about it. It would be terribly unhealthy to repress everything, pretend it didn't happen and didn't bother me, and just lock it all away. We all have things in our past we wish we would have done – or wish we never did. It's part of living and part of learning. It's not what you do, but how you see yourself while you're doing it – and after it's over – that shapes your life and determines the regrets you might have when you get older and look back over your shoulder.

The point is once you know who you are, and once you accept the idea that knowing who you are means knowing you're an addict, it's much easier to move forward from that knowledge toward what to do about it and how to live a full and rewarding life. It keeps you from staying stuck in one place or, worse yet, moving backward because you're still lost. Being an addict of any kind isn't something to just shrug off...it's a serious thing...but it's also a *reason* for past behavior that otherwise might have continued to torture you until your dying day. It helps you to understand why you've done something, so you don't have to think you're stupid, which is the most common opinion addicted people seem to have of themselves. Don't spend your life being tortured by your past like that. You have to learn, like I did, to let it go from a guilt-and-shame standpoint. I used to say – and I still believe – that you can be defeated and miserable *because of* your problems or you can be happy *in spite of* your problems. Sure, guilt and shame and all those bad feelings will still try to show up and harass you sometimes, but you can be ready for that, and well able to get through those minor setbacks and feelings that try their best to bring you to your knees just when you're learning how to stand on your own.

I haven't tried to forget my past because I use it as a good lesson for the present and the future, but I don't dwell on it either. Nothing is solved by living in the past, especially if there are few good memories back there to keep you company. I was pretty confused and lost when I first started moving toward recovery, and since I didn't know anyone else who'd been through this, I had to try and fail at some things before I found what worked for me. That's probably true of anyone who has an addiction problem, because each one of us is different and therefore must approach things in a way that works for us. One of the ways I got to this point was by looking at the people I was married to and involved with in the past and seeing the truth of the situation now instead of just what I saw through my distorted lens back then. Through that, I realized something: I didn't really wreck their lives. Sure, I might have hurt them in the past, but they – like me – have moved on from that. Some of them I still talk to, and some of them I haven't seen in years, but the Internet is an amazing tool and I can locate enough information about most of them to see that they're all right.

There are a few people, like Lee for example, who seem to be struggling, but I honestly don't feel I was the one who caused that. He had some serious problems with alcohol and other issues before I ever got involved with him, and I didn't see any evidence that his drinking had stopped the last time I saw him. I probably didn't help his situation any, but I don't think it's fair to say I did irreparable damage to him and his life, either. As for the people I married, I know a little bit about some of them and where they are today, and not so much about others. Some are easier to track down, and some have made themselves more inconspicuous, either deliberately or just by the way they live their lives. Daniel lives out west, and he works in the medical field. I don't know what his social life is like or whether he has a wife again, but at least I know he has a productive and helpful career. Beyond that information I don't know a lot about him, but there's really no reason for me to. I haven't seen him since I was eighteen, and I could probably walk right past him on the street

261

today and neither one of us would recognize the other one. We're not the same people now.

Tyler lived in a neighboring town for some time, and just recently moved away. He's remarried now, and his last job was in law enforcement. We talk occasionally, but he doesn't see his daughter much. She told him years ago she didn't want to see him anymore because he was never around when she needed him, and to my surprise he respected that. I thought for sure he'd fight it, and I'm sure it hurt him, but he accepted it and he went on with his life with his new wife and their home and their goals and dreams. He hopes for reconciliation with his daughter when she's older, and I'm leaving that up to her. I don't know what it's like to be where she is right now emotionally when it comes to her father, so I have no right to judge or to try to impress my own beliefs and opinions on her. The last I knew of Alex, he lived within an hour of me. He's remarried as well but I don't talk to him anymore, so I don't know much about his happiness level. Apparently he hadn't given up on the idea of getting married and living happily ever after, which is a good thing. I used to have a lot of ill will toward him but I don't anymore…it was only hurting me, not him.

Maximillian went through a lot of ups and downs and struggled a bit with his own identity, his spirituality, and some other problems, but he's had a good career through it all and now has a wonderful girlfriend who seems very sweet, and it appears he's finally actually happy again. He lives close by, and we still talk. I don't talk to Jack any more, but I know he's gotten married again. Where he is now, I'm not sure. I saw him one day in a store shortly after our divorce, but haven't seen him since. And then there was the man I didn't marry – Klaus. He lived near me for a long time, until some family concerns pulled him back to where he used to live. He's still single and he seems to be enjoying his time alone, but I worry about him sometimes. We're still friends, nothing more, and there won't be any backsliding where our relationship is concerned. I've changed so much I can't imagine being involved with him in a romantic way now, but I can imagine remaining his friend for many years to come. He's still struggling with his bipolar issues and sometimes he drives me crazy, but he's a good friend and a generous and happy person overall, which is more than a lot of people can say for their lives today, or for the lives of their friends – at least if they're really honest with themselves about it.

Why am I telling you all this stuff about people you've never met and likely never will? Because I'm not the only one out there like me when it comes to relationships. Because people like to have a little bit of closure in life, even if they're only reading about someone else's. Because it's important to realize the past never completely leaves us. It's part of who we are and who we will continue to become, regardless of whether we change our lifestyles, move somewhere where no one knows us, or anything else we think will give us closure or help us move on – and it's there for a reason. For me, I thought about moving away but chose to stay for the time being. I didn't want a move to be a perceived escape from my problems, and I know now that I'm capable of truly having my own life no matter where I choose to live. I'm strong enough, I have the tools I need, and I'm ready, now. If I choose to move later it will be on my terms, which is a much healthier option.

As for my other relationships – sometimes I find myself torn between not wanting to ask too much of my aging parents and wanting to make sure they still feel useful and needed. When I start to struggle with that idea I stop and take a deep breath and remind myself that my parents know I love them and they're important to me, no matter what else is taking place in my life or theirs. What better way to make them (and myself!) proud than to show them I can do things on my own, and I'll be OK after they're gone – and they won't have to worry so much. Maybe that's why they were so deeply involved with my life, because they felt they had to be and they assumed I couldn't handle things on my own. Either way, that cycle is over now. I remain close to them, emotionally, but I am building a life that belongs to *me*, now. It's based on my choices and my beliefs, not theirs or anyone else's. When I disagree with them I simply say nothing. It's much easier than fighting, it keeps the peace, and most of all it keeps *me* peaceful. It's hard to do in a way because I was so used to following their lead and working for their respect, but I have to have a life that is not dependent on others and their opinions of me for my happiness. If I don't do that, what happens to me when the others aren't there anymore? I know my parents won't always be here for me, and my daughter probably won't either. She's grown now and will want to do her own thing more and more – and *I want her to*. If she doesn't, I worry that she'll end up struggling like I did. I think she'll avoid it, largely because she's seen so much of it throughout her young life. Hopefully, she has learned from my mistakes and that will be enough to keep her from making the same ones. If I see her headed down the same path I'll speak up, but there are no guarantees she'll listen to me. People have to make their own way in life, and they can only be helped so much by those around them. Making sure I live a healthy life from now on in every way is one of the best ways to make sure my daughter does, too. I'll be leading by example, which is a good and proven way to show someone what's important in life. But she must decide what's important *for her*, and those things might not be the same as the things that I value. I have to respect that or risk repeating patterns that I want and need to avoid and remove from my life.

Being a relationship addict doesn't mean you can't have any successful, healthy relationships. It only means you have to be more careful than you might otherwise need to be. Spending time alone, and learning to enjoy your own company, is an important part of the process. The last thing you want to do is end up *needing* to be around people in order to be whole. I did that for a long time, but not anymore. I still enjoy being around other people, and I still love my parents and my daughter and the rest of my family. I still have fun with my friends, too. When they go home, or when I go back to my house after spending time with them, I'm not lonely like I used to be, and I rarely get bored any more. Someone once said only boring people get bored. I'm not sure I quite believe that, but I think there's some truth to the statement. There's always *something* to do if you're willing to go and take the time to see what interests you. I have happiness, and I have hobbies that occupy my time. I no longer think I'm a nobody unless I'm with somebody. It took me a while to get here, and I went through a lot – both good and bad – along the way, but I'm firmly here now, and the only place I'm allowing myself to go from here is forward.

It's important, if you're dealing with relationship addiction or if you know someone who is, that you see that there are others out there who are also struggling. Feeling alone in your struggle is one of the most painful things that can happen. You already feel like you need people, and then you feel like you're the only one who's in that particular predicament. It's amazing how very different – and how much better – the world looks once your opinion and understanding of your problems change. You can't 'fix' your entire life overnight, but you might be surprised how quickly you can improve things, even if you start small. Just work a little at it each day. Now that my outlook on life isn't anything like it was when I began my journey, I think it's important to talk a little bit about where I am now, to show you that there are people who *were* struggling and now are not. The contrast between where I was and where I am is something that's worth looking at. Sometimes it's amazing even to me when I take the time to look back on it.

Physically, I no longer have the widespread aches and pains I dealt with for a long time. I've 'willed them away' with prayer, meditation, and positive thinking to a large extent. I've also become more active, which has made a difference as well. It's been very difficult to do because I would get anxious every time I started to move around very much. My thoughts of having a heart problem were doing that to me, and I had to retrain my thoughts at the same time I retrained my body. I had to force myself to get some exercise and work through the anxiety, while 'talking to myself' in a positive way. The more I was able to do and not die, the better and safer I started to feel, and the more reassured I was that I really was healthy after all. What the good doctors out there were telling me was true – I did *not* have a heart *problem*, and a mildly prolapsed mitral valve was so routine and common it didn't even merit worrying about. A lot of the population have them, and the vast majority of them never cause any problem at all. While it was difficult to force myself to move when I was panicky, and it was hard to say good things to myself when my brain tried to insist I was going to just drop dead, in the end it was worth it. The positive affirmations and reassurances I said to myself every morning took a few weeks to have any effect but they did begin to help, slowly, and they seem to be gaining strength the more often and more fervently I say them. Doing something like that on a consistent basis and really believing in it can help to adjust the way you think about everything in your life.

I also gained weight. Most women would cringe at that, but I was *very* thin…like stick thin. Model thin, and it wasn't pretty. It might look good on sixteen and seventeen-year-old models on the catwalk, but it doesn't look so good on an average-looking, late-thirties woman out in the real world. People asked if I was ill; they thought I was anorexic, or maybe I was incredibly poor and didn't have enough money for food. I bought my clothing from the juniors department because nothing else fit, and the clothes I'd worn before I married Jack were literally falling off me. I knew I had to do something, but I just couldn't eat. I felt too bad to care, and nothing sounded good. As I slowly started to get my life straightened out I started to feel better and started to have more of an appetite, so I took advantage of that to deliberately gain a little bit of weight. I'm still thin, and I plan to stay that way, but gaining just a few pounds gave me more energy, more stamina, and better general health. It also helped to reduce the number of skipped heartbeats I was getting as well as the episodes of racing heartbeat and dizziness. My panic attacks lessened. It lifted my overall mood, which I found pleasantly surprising. Those simple things along with a better diet and some light exercise have helped me to feel much healthier than I did in the past.

Emotionally, I'm also healthier. Now that I don't just know but also *understand* the real issue behind the struggles and problems I've had I can be a work in progress instead of just stagnating where I was. Admitting to an addiction can be a humbling experience, but also a freeing one. It's not an *excuse* for what I did, but it *is* a reason, and that helps to settle the other struggle I've had – the one with guilt and shame. It's still there, but it's lessened by the realization that there was a reason why I kept doing what I was doing – I wasn't stupid. I have a legitimate problem which I'm now dealing with. It will be with me throughout the rest of my life, but that doesn't mean it has to *control* the rest of my life. Being able to accept that and embrace it has definitely helped my outlook on life overall and made me much more comfortable in my own skin. I have fewer panic attacks and I'm hopeful that my anxiety will go into complete remission again. If it doesn't, I'm better prepared to deal with it now, and I don't see it as being as much of a burden as I used to, mostly because a lot of the other emotional burdens I was wrestling with have been removed or at least greatly reduced. My past struggles with anxiety are just part of who I am, and I'm not ashamed of it. It's another one of those thing that just *is*; another issue that requires acceptance and understanding in order to see improvement.

Then there's the issue of spirituality. I'd have to say I'm much farther along in my spiritual journey than I thought I'd ever be, but of course there's still a long way to go. When I started on that path I did so because of a desire to have peace and contentment, yes, but I also did it because Klaus was doing it and it was something new for me – more drama. At first it was exciting and mystic and I made a big deal out of it. Now I don't say much about it. It's become *real* to me, another part of who I am, instead of just a point of high drama in my life. I see it as something that *matters*, now, and because of that I don't have the need to go and tell everyone I meet all about it. I realize I'm telling you about it here, but that has a point to it. I'm not running up to strangers on the street and 'being spiritual' at them anymore. I'm no longer looking for acceptance from others because I have it from myself and from God, and that's really all I require. I do believe people need others, though. No man is an island, and all that. Still, I think there's a difference between needing people in that you want to be around them and enjoy their company, and needing people in that you can't be *you* without *them*. I used to belong to the second category, and now I belong to the first. I feel like I've been released from prison, and in a way I guess I have, at least emotionally. I knew where the lock was all that time, and I just had to find the key.

I can honestly say I don't know anyone else whose life-changing spiritual transformation has been brought about by German hip-hop music – maybe my daughter to some extent, but mostly I think she's always been interested in spirituality and afraid to show it until I did. Where the music is concerned, I may be unique in that respect. The music was what started my whole journey, but it wasn't something that was a catalyst and then disappeared. I still listen to it, and I always will. Not a day goes by when I'm not either playing music or at least hearing it in my head. But I've heard a lot of different stories about strange and amazing things that changed people's lives, and based on some of those I might not be so different after all. There are all kinds of things that can have a profound impact on our lives.

Some of them are huge, like marriages and cross-country moves and children being born and then growing up to have children of their own, and the death of relatives. These are the kinds of things no one ever forgets; all seemingly unavoidable parts of our lives and the lives of everyone around us. But what about all the little things that have an impact on us? We see a butterfly in the yard and it makes us smile, or we get an unexpected sunny day during a predicted rainy weekend, or we receive an email from a friend we haven't heard from in years. Or maybe we hear of the loss of a colleague but we don't have time to stop and mourn properly – there's always so much to do. So many things happen to us each day, and we don't even *notice* them. We're too busy; focused on our jobs, our families, our so-called lives. But we're not really living by doing things that way. We're only playing a role and going through the motions of life. We're not fully in the moment, and since we don't even realize it, we can't change it.

Most people live their whole lives that way. I was one of the lucky ones…all the problems I went through were well worth the joy and awareness I have now. I see the beauty in life and the importance of it; that everyone and everything has a value and a purpose, even if it's hard to see what that might be at the time. I see how much joy is out there, and it's all mine – all I have to do is go get it. You might say you don't know how to do that. Of course you do! Just go and do what makes you happy. Embrace the things that bring you joy. If you don't remember what those things are any more, maybe it's time for some soul-searching. Those things haven't been lost to you even if you can't think of them right now. They'll come back to you…and you might find others to add in along the way. It doesn't have to be anything expensive or fancy. Just something that brings beauty to your life or to the lives of others. I'll give you an example from my own life – something that's so simple, something that doesn't cost much, something that never fails to lift my mood and make me smile. Butterflies.

Near where I live there is a 'butterfly house.' It's closed during the winter, and it only opens up during certain days in the summer. They take donations to stay open, and it's just a small little place, but it's interesting and fun. If you go there, like I often do when it's closed and quiet, you can find butterflies outside in the trees and bushes. They're all over the place. The only thing it costs me is the gasoline to get there, and it takes less than five minutes so it doesn't add up to much. When the monarchs come through on their annual migration, the trees are covered in them. If you reach up gently you can slide your hand under these delicate, winged creatures and pluck them off the shrubbery. They'll walk around on you until they figure out you're not a flower, and then they'll flit back to the trees until you pluck them off again. As long as you're careful you don't hurt them, and they're not capable of hurting you. It's a way to commune with nature, and it's almost meditative as you study these gentle insects. The trees and flowers smell good, and the movement of the butterflies' wings fans that fragrance to you. It's incredibly peaceful. Maybe you don't like butterflies and nature and trees and flowers as much as I do. That's OK. There are literally millions of simple, inexpensive things you can do to make you joyful and then you can carry that joy around and give it away to others.

I'm not the only one who has had the privilege of finding joy in simple things, and in just being alive to appreciate how much beauty and love are really out there. Addictions can be difficult and painful and debilitating, sure, but they can also be life-changing and affirming. Here's another example of a seemingly simple thing to be joyous about: I once heard a woman say she was so glad she was an alcoholic – if she hadn't gone through everything the disease entailed and then had an intervention and gotten sober, there's so much she would've missed out on. At her lowest point she was drinking heavily and taking medication for bipolar disorder – and way too much medication, too; more than she needed and more than she'd been prescribed. She could have easily killed herself – just gone to sleep and never woken up – but she really didn't want to die. She described how her brother found her and called the paramedics because he couldn't wake her. She was so angry with him for doing that; from the detox facility she said she hated him and she never wanted to speak to him again. How could he have done this to her? Now they are closer than ever, and she's been sober for years. She also gained something else – an appreciation for life now that she probably never would've attained if she'd not been through those bad times. You appreciate the beauty of the light so much more when you come to it out of the darkness.

Whether it's you or someone you love who's dealing with relationship addiction, it's important to not only see that others share that pain, but that recovery and moving forward are possible. I want others to know they can get help, and they can also help themselves. That's the main thing so many people with addiction problems either don't realize or don't truly believe in, so I'll say it again – *you can help yourself.* If you feel you need to seek professional help with your addiction, there is absolutely nothing wrong with that. Don't feel bad about seeking help. Many people do, and even more people *should* but never do. Even if you do that, know that a therapist can't 'fix' you…he or she can only help you understand your problems and give you tools and resources you can use to adjust and control your behavior. These are important things, but they're not the same as a 'cure.' In other words, you still have to do the work yourself, and you have to be committed to that work or it won't get done. If you're able to understand and address your issues on your own, there's nothing wrong with that, either.

The only thing I would say as a cautionary statement for people who choose to avoid traditional therapy is that it's very easy to say you can handle it (or are handling it) on your own when in fact that's not really the case. Don't let that become an excuse – which you see as a reason – not to go to a therapist or get actual help some other way. You have to be honest with yourself not just about your past, but about your present and future as well. If you just say you can handle it and that's why you aren't going to therapy and yet you actually do nothing, you're not just hurting yourself. You're also hurting the people who rely on you and the people who care about you and the people who believe in you. Even if you don't matter much to yourself, I'll bet those other people matter to you. And you matter to them, as well. If you won't get help or start helping yourself *for you*, then please find someone or something that matters to you, and do it for *them*. In time, as you start to feel better, you'll start doing it for yourself – but the important thing is that you get started. Nothing will happen on its own to just magically make it better. I know. I waited a long time for that to take place, but nothing changed. It was only when I took a deep breath and dove in that good things started happening.

Whether your path lies through professional help or through self-discovery and spiritual growth, or whether it's some combination of the two, it's very important to know there is *always* hope, no matter how dark the circumstances seem at the time. You can say it's hopeless, and you can even really mean it, but it's not actually true. It's something your brain tells you, not your soul – much like the way my brain would try to tell me I was having a heart attack when it was just my anxiety. You don't have to have anxiety or even depression problems in order to have your brain mislead you. I think it happens to everyone to some extent, but some of us are more susceptible than others. It comes from brain chemistry, but also from how you were raised and what shaped your childhood. If you can learn to trust your gut – your heart, your soul, your spirit, whatever term you choose to use – instead of only ever trusting what your brain and your thoughts tell you, you can do a lot more and feel a lot better...and I don't mean don't think about what you're doing. You still have to live like a rational human being and we have brains for a reason – but be sure the thoughts you're thinking are *the right thoughts*. Be sure they're true and honest and realistic and not just something you're telling yourself to remain in denial.

This is something it took me a long time to learn, but once I learned it – really *learned* it and internalized it – I've found it never leaves me. I still get anxious, depressed, lonely, and all of those things sometimes, but not like I used to. Everyone gets that way sometimes. When I do feel that way I know how to look at it now, and I know how to deal with it. That understanding makes all the difference. Where I go from here is something I really *can* control – as much as anyone can control his or her own destiny – because of the awareness I've developed. I also know there are people out there who've been married more times than I have, or who've had many far worse experiences. Some of these people have been mistreated by their parents or by their spouses, or they've been the long-term victims of what seems to be a lot of bad luck. Some people just can't seem to get a break and it seems like, no matter what they do, they're always somehow struggling with things that appear to be beyond their control. I don't ever mean to make light of the plight of people like this, and I don't mean for the information in this book to come across as though I think nobody has ever had it worse than me. It's not intended as a sob story. It's intended to show that relationship addiction is real, and it's not something that should be ignored any longer.

Because a lot of people don't know about it it's still not well understood, and when you mention it to most people you have to stop and explain what it is. I've done that before, and I've gotten some funny looks from people who I thought would 'get it.' I've also gotten some really interesting conversations from people who I thought wouldn't understand at all. It turns out they do understand – and they know someone like that, too. Brothers, sisters, parents, and friends, it seems like more and more people can tell stories of people they know who are having problems with the relationships around them. Overall, I find I end up explaining the term quite a lot. People understand the symptoms because they see them, but they don't know there's a term for it; that it's really called something, and that there's a way their friends and relatives can get some help for it. They think, like I did for so long, that it's just something that's happening through bad choices, and there's no actual *reason* for it to be taking place.

Seeing how many people reflect that opinion tells me more knowledge of relationship addiction should be out there, in order to help more struggling people. Individuals who don't know much about it can't help themselves, and they can't help others who might need them. They don't understand what's happening to their lives and why things seem so out of control. They don't know they're addicts and accepting and understanding that can help them take their first steps toward a better life for themselves and the people who care for them – and they need to be told, as clearly as possible and as often as possible until it clicks for them. It's not something they'll probably accept the first time they hear it – I know I certainly didn't.

Instead, they have to be reminded in a way they're comfortable with. If you order someone to 'straighten up' you're just setting yourself up for rebellion. They have to come to an understanding of the issue on their own terms and that doesn't come from being ordered around. It comes from caring and compassion and persistence. Once a person is willing to accept something and be accountable for it the real work begins, but so do the real rewards, and those are worth every struggle to get to them. As for me, I've come to terms with what I've done and why I did it, and I really am content and at peace with it, now. How I got there might not work for everyone, but I *did* get there, and I want to be sure others know they can get there, too. That's why I tell my story and why I'll continue to do so, as often as I can, to anyone who genuinely wants to listen. The journey is far from over.

What The Therapist Says

Many people have very specific ideas about what they wish to accomplish when they set out to deal with their codependency and relationship issues. Often their goals center on wanting to be able to finally have a "good" relationship. Others wish to achieve independence from partners, parents, or even children. It does not really matter what goal the codependent relationship addict has in mind when first making those tentative steps toward self-improvement. Most methods will, sooner or later, focus the sufferer's attention on themselves – mainly, on who they really are. But awareness of what our "self" is only represents the first step in an amazing journey of self-discovery.

To know who we are is essential, but not enough to live a fulfilled life. What good is it to be aware of our identity if we really do not like it? Hence, learning to love the "self" is the most important aspect of healing those deep-rooted self-worth problems underlying codependency and the addictive behaviors it gives rise to. In hindsight it may seem ironic that such a lofty goal, being able to love oneself unconditionally, can be achieved with rather simple steps. Often we seek a wondrous insight or divine revelation that will cure everything that ails us. In reality the means to our recovery are often minute, everyday techniques. And they do not require special skills or insight. What they do require is practice and continuous usage. Brushing one's teeth is not complicated. But we have to do it every day in order to have healthy teeth.

Affirmations, practicing stopping and re-directing our thoughts, counting things that we are grateful for, all of these small methods can have a huge impact if engaged in regularly. So what kind of self-help regimen do I espouse? That is a difficult question, not in terms of what I personally do to keep my self-esteem healthy, and I have to actively "keep" it healthy just like everyone else, but as far as what will help others. The bottom line is that since everyone's issues with self-worth are different, each person will respond better to a different "menu" of selected self-improvement techniques. As this chapter comes to a close, I would like to list some of my personal favorites and those my clients have found most helpful:

1.) Self-affirmations: Finding time to, either in front of a mirror or by oneself, tell ourselves out loud that we like ourselves. Or, finding specific things we can point out about ourselves that are likable.

2.) Gratitude lists: Starting the day by listing a number of things we are grateful for. A set number – five, ten, fifteen – helps to keep the practice regimented. This starts the day and our subconscious off on a positive note.

3.) Disengage criticism / Nevertheless method: Whenever we receive criticism, be it from others or ourselves, make sure to re-phrase the criticism in a way that separates our actions from our worth: "I have done something wrong, *nevertheless* I am a worthwhile person."

4.) Here and now focus: When we feel trapped in our worries about the future, past, or what people may think of us, focus the mind on the here and now. Use your senses to focus your attention on a sight, sound, smell, anything that fills you with enjoyment.

5.) Artistic expression: Music, art, poetry, either appreciated or produced can be a great outlet for those deeply-held emotions we would be afraid to express otherwise.

6.) Meditation / Prayer: Finding a means of mentally disconnecting with our worries through some relaxation exercise or mantra. Much of our addictive behaviors are release mechanisms for emotional pressure that can also be released through meditative practices.

7.) Support groups: You are not alone. Sometimes just seeing that other people go through similar hardships can help ease the isolation of codependent suffering. Plus, as one sees that others suffering from similar concerns are still worthwhile people, one can begin to accept the possibility than one is maybe not as worthless as previously thought.

8.) Professional help: Seeking the aid of a therapist can be very helpful. Sometimes an outside perspective, especially if coupled with a sense of authority (the subconscious loves authority) can help us derail our old self-defeating habits of thought.

9.) Medication: There are measurable medical conditions that affect our moods and perspectives. Bipolar disorder, anxiety disorders, clinical depression, obsessive-compulsive disorder, and others often have a true physiological component that requires medicinal intervention.

Which of these venues a sufferer from relationship addiction wishes to try is up to personal preference. Many times a codependent will go through different phases in his or her life, utilizing one method and then switching to another as recovery progresses. There is no "best way" to seek healing for our innermost self. Many times the honest desire and making that first step in engaging in a method aimed at dealing with the demon of codependence is the hardest. Sometimes it is not. In most cases the recovery process will take time. Habits that have taken a lifetime to learn are not likely to be undone in a single day.

On the other hand they also do not require an equal amount of time to be remedied. A good friend of mine began his recovery journey at age 85 and has now, two and a half years later, reached a point in his life that he never believed possible. He is happy and content now, after more than eight decades of being depressed. Whenever one of my clients or I get overcome by hopelessness, I remind myself of my friend. Whether recovery is possible depends mostly on one thing – our desire and dedication to try and work on it.

The rewards for taking this daring leap into the unknown are difficult to describe. As the reader might have guessed, I myself have traveled this road. I can honestly say that the recovery process, as frightening and overwhelming as it may seem at times, leads to a sense of serenity, a word I do not use lightly, that I could not have previously imagined. Does it lead to a state of perfect bliss? Of course not! Life will still have its ups and downs. Relationships may fail. What will change is how we will be able to deal with it and still feel that we are good and worthwhile.

Codependence causes people to worry so much about others and what they might think. It makes one crave a million external means to validate oneself, all measured on scales of success learned through childhood that we are not even aware of in our conscious minds. It is remarkable that in this process and all the addictions that grow from it the sufferer disregards one opinion and validation the most: his or her own "self." Learning to love the "self" is a concept almost alien to our culture. If we do not produce we are not worthy. If we do not have we are nothing. The one thing that should be the easiest thing to do for anyone has become unbearably hard in today's culture: we have lost the skill to simply "be," and to be happy doing just that.

For all those who have seen some of their own lives reflected in the author's journey, for those who have realized their own desire to grow out of old chains of thought and behavior, I want to encourage you to take that first step. It is a worthwhile journey to make. No matter what you may currently believe about yourself, your abilities, your character, or your innate value, you deserve love, happiness and prosperity. Everyone does, no matter whether they believe it or not. My deepest wish for all those who have read this book is to find these things, and accept them when they have been found.

Chapter 12: Resources to Help Your Recovery

Not everyone responds to recovery in the same way, and not everyone will be helped in the same way. For that reason, the resources presented here cover various types of addiction and self-esteem issues and focus on everything from first-person accounts to clinical workbooks. A reader can take what works for him from this list as he starts on his own journey of recovery.

- *Relationship/Love/Sex Addiction & Codependency*
<u>Books</u>
Carnes, Patrick J. *Don't Call It Love*. New York: Bantam Books, 1991.
Carnes, Patrick J. *Certification in Sexual Addiction Workshop Manual:* October 9-13, 2000.
Fromm, Erich. *The Art of Loving*. New York: Harper and Row, 1962.
Karen, Robert. *Becoming Attached: First Relationships and How They Shape Our Capacity to Love*. New York: Oxford University Press, 1998.
Lewis, Thomas, Amini, Fari and Lannon, Richard. *A General Theory of Love*. New York: Vintage Books, 2000.
Mellody, Pia. *Facing Love Addiction: Giving Yourself the Power to Change the Way You Love*. San Francisco: Harper Collins, 1992.
Sbraga, Tamara Penix and O'Donohue, William T. *The Sex Addiction Workbook*. Oakland, California: New Harbinger Publications, 2003.
Schaef, Anne Wilson. *When Society Becomes an Addict*. San Francisco: Harper and Row, 1987.
Schaef, Anne Wilson. *Escape from Intimacy: Untangling the "Love Addictions: Sex, Romance, and Relationships*. San Francisco: Harper San Francisco, 1990.
Schaeffer, Brenda. *Is It Love or Is It Addiction?* Center City, Minnesota: Hazelden, 1987.
Schaeffer, Brenda. *Loving Me, Loving You: Balancing Love and Power in a Codependent World*. Center City, Minnesota: Hazelden, 1991.

Wile, Daniel B. *After the Fight: Using your Disagreements to Build a Stronger Relationship.* New York: The Guilford Press, 1993.

Articles
Carnes, Patrick J., Murray, Robert E., Charpentier, Louis. "Bargains with Chaos: Sex Addicts and Interaction Disorder." *Sexual Addiction & Compulsivity,* 12:79-120, 2005.
Goodman, Aviel. "Diagnosis and Treatment of Sexual Addiction." *Journal of Sex & Marital Therapy*, 19, 3, 225-251, Fall 1993.

Websites
About Love Addiction – http://www.recovery-man.com/loveaddict.htm
Codependents Anonymous – http://www.codependents.org
Mental Health America: Codependency – http://www.nmha.org/go/codependency
On Love Addiction – http://love-addiction.com/onlove.html
Relationship Addict – http://relationshipaddict.com/
Self-Esteem and Codependency Self-Exam – http://www.casaesperanza.org/resources/selfassess_E.cfm
Sex Addicts Anonymous – http://www.sexaa.org
Sex and Love Addicts Anonymous – http://www.slaawfs.org

▪ **Self Esteem and Self-Help**
Books
Benson, Herbert. *The Relaxation Response.* New York: William Morrow and Co., 1975.
Bilodeau, Lorrainne. *The Anger Workbook.* Center City, Minnesota: Hazelden, 1992.
King, Serge Kalihi. *Mastering Your Hidden Self: A Guide to The Huna Way.* Wheaton, Illinois: Quest Books, 1985.
Long, Max Freedom. *Self-Suggestion and The New Huna Theory of Mesmerism and Hypnosis.* Los Angeles: De Vorrs, 1958.

Ray, Sondra. *I Deserve Love: How Affirmations Can Guide You to Personal Fulfillment.* Millbrae, California: Les Femmes, 1976.

Ruskan, John. *Emotional Clearing: A Self-Therapy Guide to Releasing Negative Feelings.* New York: R. Wyler and Company, 1993.

Websites
National Mental Health Information Center: Self-Esteem Activities –
http://mentalhealth.samhsa.gov/publications/allpubs/sma-3715/activities.asp
Life 123: Stress Management –
http://www.life123.com/health/stress-management/index.shtml
Meditation Handbook –
http://home.att.net/~meditation/MeditationHandbook.html

- *Alcohol & Drug Addiction*
Books
Alcoholics Anonymous World Services. *Alcoholics Anonymous,* Fourth Edition. New York, 2001.

Brown, Stephanie. *Treating the Alcoholic: A Developmental Model of Recovery.* New York: John Wiley & Sons, 1985.

Brown, Stefanie and Yalom, Irvin, Editors. *Treating Alcoholism.* San Francisco: Jossey-Bass, 1995.

Brown, Stefanie and Lewis, Virginia. *The Alcoholic Family in Recovery.* New York: The Guilford Press, 1999.

Dardis, Tom. *The Thirsty Muse: Alcohol and the American Writer.* New York: Ticknor & Fields, 1989.

Gorski, Terence and Miller, Merlene. *Staying Sober: A Guide for Relapse Prevention.* Independence, Missouri: Independence Press, 1986.

Hamill, Pete. *A Drinking Life: A Memoir.* New York: Back Bay Books, 1995.

Hayle, Aletha. *Opium and the Romantic Imagination.* Berkeley, California: University of California Press, 1968.

Inaba, Darryl S. and Cohen, William E. *Uppers, Downers, All Arounders.* Ashland, Oregon: CNS Publications, Inc., Fourth Edition, 2000.

Knapp, Caroline. *Drinking: A Love Story.* New York: Dial Press, 1997.

Margolis, Robert D. and Zweben, Joan E. *Treating Patients with Alcohol and Other Drug Problems: An Integrated Approach.* Washington, D.C.: American Psychological Association, 1998.

Miller, William R. and Munoz, Ricardo F. *Controlling Your Drinking.* New York: The Guilford Press, 2005.

Miller, William R. and Carroll, Kathleen M. *Rethinking Substance Abuse: What the Science Shows, and What We Should Do About It.* New York: The Guilford Press, 2006.

Nicolaus, Martin. *Recovery by Choice: Living and Enjoying life Free of Alcohol and Drugs: A Workbook.* Oakland, CA: LifeRing Press,Third Printing, 2006.

Schuckit, Marc A. *Educating Yourself About Alcohol and Drugs: A People's Primer.* New York: Plenum Press, 1995.

Vaillant, George E. *The Natural History of Alcoholism Revisited,* Harvard University Press, Cambridge, MA; 1995.

Washton, Arnold M. and Zweben, Joan E. *Treating Alcohol and Drug Problems in Psychotherapy Practice: Doing What Works.* New York: The Guilford Press, 2006.

Articles

Davis, Diane Rae and Jansen, Golie G. "Making Meaning of Alcoholics Anonymous for Social Workers: Myths, Metaphors, and Realities." *Social Work,* 43,2, 169-182, March, 1998.

Kaskutas, Lee Ann and Oberste, Edward. "Making Alcoholics Anonymous Easier: A Manual." Alcohol Research Group, *Public Health Institute,* 2002.

Matano, Robert A. and Yalom, Irvin D. "Approaches to Chemical Dependency: Chemical Dependency and Interactive Group Therapy – A Synthesis." *International Journal of Group Psychotherapy,* 41, 3, 269-293, 1991.

Witkiewitz, Katie and Marlatt, G. Alan. "Relapse Prevention for Alcohol and Drug problems: That Was Zen, This Is Tao." *American Psychologist*, 59, 4, 224-235, May-June 2004.

Wood, M., Read, J., Mitchell, R. and Brand, N. "Do Parents Still Matter? Parent and Peer Influences on Alcohol Involvement Among Recent High School Graduates." *Psychology of Addictive Behaviors*, 18,1, 19-30, 2004.

Websites

Alcoholics Anonymous – http://www.alcoholics-anonymous.org

Love Addicts Anonymous – http://loveaddicts.org/index.html

MedlinePlus – http://www.nlm.nih.gov/medlineplus/news/fullstory_65708.html

National Institute on Chemical Dependency – http://www.nicd.us/familyresources.html

Online AA Recovery Resources – http://www.recovery.org/aa/

- ▪ *Other Addiction Resources*

Books

Biglan, A., Brennan, P.A., Foster, S. L., Holder, H.D. *Helping Adolescents at Risk: Prevention of Multiple Problem Behaviors*. New York: The Guilford Press, 2004.

Bradshaw, John. *Bradshaw On: Healing the Shame That Binds You*. Deerfield, Florida: Health Communications, Inc., 1988.

Carnes, Patrick J. *The Betrayal Bond*. Deerfield Beach, Florida: Health Communications, Inc., 1997.

Carnes, Patrick J. *A Gentle Path through the Twelve Steps*. Center City, Minnesota: Hazelden, 1993.

Denning, Patt. *Practicing Harm Reduction Psychotherapy: An Alternative Approach to Addictions*. New York: The Guilford Press, 2000.

DiClemente, Carlo. *Addiction and Change: How Addictions Develop and Addicted People Recover*. New York: Guilford Press, 2006.

Fanning, Patrick, and John Terence O'Neill. *The Addiction Workbook*. New York: New Harbinger Press, 1996.

Howard, Pierce J. *The Owner's Manual for the Brain: Everyday Applications from Mind-Brain Research,* Third Edition. Austin, TX: Bard Press, 2006.

Kendler, Kenneth S. and Prescott, Carol A. *Genes, Environment, and Psychopathology*. New York: The Guilford Press, 2006.

Linehan, Marsha M. *Cognitive-Behavioral Treatment of Borderline Personality Disorder*. New York: The Guilford Press, 1993.

Marlatt, G. Alan and Gordon, Judith R. *Relapse Prevention*. New York: The Guilford Press, 1985.

Masterson, James F. *The Real Self: A Developmental, Self, and Object Relations Approach*. New York: Brunner/Mazel Publishers, 1985.

Nakken, Craig. *The Addictive Personality*. St. Paul, Minnesota: Hazelden, 1996.

Zuckerman, Marvin. *Sensation Seeking and Risky Behavior.* Washington, D.C.: American Psychological Association, 2007.

Articles

Anda, R.F., Felitti, V.J. "Adverse Childhood Experiences and their Importance to Adult Health and Well-being." *Congressional Briefing*. April 18, 2006.

Brody, Jane E. "A Revolution at 50: Personal Health; Genes may Draw Your Road Map, But You Can Still Chart Your Course." *The New York Times*, nytimes.com, February 25, 2003.

Denizet-Lewis, Benoit. "An Anti-Addiction Pill?" *The New York Times Magazine*, June 25, 48-53, 2006.

Dube, S.R., Felitti,V.J., Dong, M., Chapman, D.P., Giles, W.H., Anda, R.F. "Childhood Abuse, Neglect, and Household Dysfunction and the Risk of Illicit Drug Use: The Adverse Childhood Experiences Study." *Pediatrics,* 111, 564-572 2003.

Felitti, V.J., Anda, R.F., Nordenberg, D., Williamson, D.F., Spitz, A.M., Edwards, V., Koss, M.P., Marks, J.S. "Relationship of Childhood Abuse and Household Dysfunction to Many of the Leading Causes of Death in

Adults." *American Journal of Preventive Medicine*, 14 (4): 245-258, 1998.

Felitti,V.J. "The Origins of Addictions: Evidence from the Adverse Childhood Experiences Study." English version of the article published in Germany as: Ursprunge des Suchtverhaltens- Evidenzen aus einer Studie zu belastenden Kindheitserfahrungen. *Praxis der Kinderpsychologie und Kinderpsychiatrie*, 52:547-559, 2003.

Guisinger, Shan and Blatt, J. Sidney J. "Individuality and Relatedness: Evolution of a Fundamental Dialectic." *American Psychologist*, 49, 2, 104-111, February 1994.

Leshner, Alan L. "Addiction is a Brain Disease, and It Matters." *Science*, 278, 45-47,1997.

Robinson, Terry E. & Berridge, Kent C. "Addiction." *Annual Review of Psychology*, 54, 25-53, 2003.

Shaffer, Howard J., LaPlante, Debi A., LaBrie, Richard A., Kidman, Rachel C., Donato, Anthony N., and Stanton, Michael V. "Toward a Syndrome Model of Addiction: Multiple Expressions, Common Etiology." *Harvard Review of Psychiatry*, 12: 367-364, 2004.

Whitfield, C.L. "Adverse Childhood Experiences and Trauma." *American Journal of Preventive Medicine*, 14 (4): 361-364,1998.

Websites

About Addictions and Addicts – http://www.topaddictions.com/
Internet, Porn, and Cybersex Addictions –
http://www.helpguide.org/mental/internet_cybersex_
addiction.htm

9 781849 915168